Risky Alcohol Consumption among Adolescents

Silke Diestelkamp • Rainer Thomasius

Risky Alcohol Consumption among Adolescents

Manual for the Implementation of a Brief Motivational Intervention

With Contributions by Katrin Lammers and Udo J. Küstner

Springer

Silke Diestelkamp
University Clinic Hamburg-Eppendorf
German Center for Addiction Research in Childhood and Adolescence
Hamburg, Hamburg, Germany

Rainer Thomasius
University Clinic Hamburg-Eppendorf
German Center for Addiction Research in Childhood and Adolescence
Hamburg, Hamburg, Germany

ISBN 978-3-662-68634-8 ISBN 978-3-662-68635-5 (eBook)
https://doi.org/10.1007/978-3-662-68635-5

This book is a translation of the original German edition „Riskanter Alkoholkonsum bei Jugendlichen" by Diestelkamp, Silke, published by Springer-Verlag GmbH, DE in 2017. The translation was done with the help of artificial intelligence (machine translation by the service DeepL.com). A subsequent human revision was done primarily in terms of content, so that the book will read stylistically differently from a conventional translation. Springer Nature works continuously to further the development of tools for the production of books and on the related technologies to support the authors.

This book is a translation of the original German edition "Riskanter Alkoholkonsum bei Jugendlichen" by Silke Diestelkamp et al., published by Springer-Verlag GmbH, DE in 2017. The translation was done with the help of an artificial intelligence machine translation tool. A subsequent human revision was done primarily in terms of content, so that the book will read stylistically differently from a conventional translation. Springer Nature works continuously to further the development of tools for the production of books and on the related technologies to support the authors.

This Springer imprint is published by the registered company Springer-Verlag GmbH, DE, part of Springer Nature.
The registered company address is: Heidelberger Platz 3, 14197 Berlin, Germany

Foreword

The project HaLT—Hart am LimiT was developed by the "Villa Schöpflin", a foundation-funded addiction prevention facility in Lörrach, in 2002. Due to the steady increase in the number of cases of alcohol-intoxicated children and adolescents, the Federal Ministry of Health funded a pilot phase in Lörrach from 2003 to 2004. After the successful start, the project was promoted in 2007 as a federal model project at ten further locations in nine federal states. In the meantime, HaLT—Hart am LimiT exists in 14 federal states at a total of 155 locations. The initiators of HaLT—Hart am LimiT have always advocated a holistic prevention approach with proactive and reactive components. HaLT—Hart am LimiT should not only focus on alcohol-intoxicated children and adolescents, but should conceptually include universal and selective prevention. At the time when we decided on the project, Hamburg already had a structurally distinctive alcohol prevention, so that only the reactive component of HaLT—Hart am LimiT was missing in the multitude of offers. Initially, the bedside interventions were carried out by employees of an addiction counselling centre. At that time, funding was provided exclusively through grants. Since 2011, thanks to a joint framework agreement with the statutory health insurance funds and the associated financial support, we have been able to carry out the project at six Hamburg hospitals with trained professionals on weekend days (Friday to Sunday). Currently, eight trained freelance specialists go to the hospitals and carry out the intervention at the hospital bedside under the supervision of the supra-regional Addiction Counselling Centre for Adolescents Kö16a. However, a randomised-controlled evaluation of the effectiveness of this brief motivational intervention at the hospital bedside has not yet been carried out. Against this background, the Hamburg participants decided to develop the HaLT Hamburg Manual and the associated training. Within the framework of the psychenet research network, the German Centre for Addiction Research in Childhood and Adolescence (DZSKJ) obtained research funding from the Federal Ministry of Education and Research (BMBF) and used it to implement an effectiveness study of HaLT-Hamburg and to produce the present manual. With the scientific expertise of the DZSKJ, the practical experience of Katrin Lammers (Kö16) and that of Udo Küstner (Drug and Alcohol Outpatient Clinic for Adolescents, Young Adults and their Families at the University Medical Center Hamburg-Eppendorf), it was possible to develop this comprehensive manual for brief intervention, with which we can contribute to the further development of brief motivational interventions at the bedside nationwide. It is a good example of interdisciplinary cooperation and successful science-practice transfer. We would like to thank the UKE, Professor Thomasius, Ms. Diestelkamp, Mr. Arnaud and Mr. Küstner.

Sven Kammerahl
Department of Drugs and Addiction, Ministry of Health and Consumer Protection of the Free and Hanseatic City of Hamburg, Hamburg, Germany

Foreword

The prevention programme HaLT—Hart am LimiT stands for quality-assured prevention for the prevention of youth alcohol abuse throughout Germany. The uniqueness and success of this programme, which was developed in 2002 by Villa Schöpflin gGmbH—Centre for Addiction Prevention in Lörrach, lies in the combination of behavioural and relationship prevention measures. In the past years, a network of 155 locations in 14 federal states has developed with this successful model.

The behavioural prevention measures form the "reactive component" of HaLT. The core of this component is addressing young people who have been hospitalised due to alcohol intoxication. On the basis of motivational interviewing, they and their parents receive an individually tailored offer of help. This indicated prevention offer is complemented by a prevention strategy anchored in the community, the "proactive component". By involving regional actors from various professions, harmful alcohol consumption among young people is to be prevented. Consistent compliance with the protection of minors plays a central role here.

The HaLT programme is continuously scientifically monitored and further developed as part of quality assurance. Since November 2014, this has been ensured by the HaLT Service Center, which was founded specifically for this purpose and is financed by the Schöpflin Foundation. The Service Center coordinates central activities in the HaLT network nationwide, guarantees regular training for professionals, provides the network with up-to-date materials and information, and represents the programme at the political level.

HaLT—Hart am LimiT has been implemented in Hamburg since 2007 and is one of the largest locations nationwide. In the implementation of both components, the Hamburg location has a nationwide exemplary character. In the reactive component, excellent cooperation has developed with six Hamburg clinics as well as with the German Centre for Addiction Research in Childhood and Adolescence. These cooperations enabled the scientific monitoring of the Hamburg location in the form of a study, which forms the basis of this manual. The subject of the study was the effectiveness and feasibility of the previous HaLT brief intervention in hospitals. On this empirical basis, this valid tool for the implementation of the brief intervention for adolescents with risky alcohol consumption has now been developed. As a supplement to the HaLT manual of Villa Schöpflin gGmbH, the Hamburg manual can be recommended to all HaLT prevention specialists in the federal network.

Susanne Schmitt
HaLT Service Center of the Schöpflin Foundation, Lörrach, Germany

Preface

Risky alcohol consumption in adolescence is widespread and for many young people a temporary phenomenon from which they grow out "on their own" as they get older. But can we therefore trivialise risky consumption at this age? We would like to give an example of an encounter in the winter of 2010/2011. We sat down with Prof. Püschel, the director of the Department of Forensic Medicine at the University Medical Center Hamburg-Eppendorf, to discuss a project idea. When we reported on the HaLT Hamburg study, which was about to begin, Prof. Püschel told us about two young girls he recently had to autopsy. Both girls had—independently of each other—frozen to death at night in front of discotheques because they had fallen asleep in the snow or slipped into a ditch while heavily intoxicated. They had gone outside lightly dressed because the queues in front of the toilets were too long for them. Excessive alcohol consumption can have serious consequences, even when drinking infrequently.

This is why the prevention programme HaLT—Hart am LimiT developed by the Addiction Prevention Centre Villa Schöpflin is so important, as it is not only aimed at the small group of young people with a possible addiction risk, but also at the large group of young people who potentially put themselves and others at risk through episodic excessive alcohol consumption. The "reactive component" of this project is aimed at children and adolescents who are being treated in a clinic due to acute alcohol intoxication and has the goal of motivating these particularly at-risk children and adolescents in a counselling session to low-risk consumption or abstinence.

The effectiveness of this approach has now been investigated in the randomised-controlled HaLT-Hamburg study. The study was part of the joint project *psychenet*—Hamburg Network for Mental Health, which consists of more than 80 Hamburg scientific and medical institutions, counselling centres, the Senate and Chamber of Commerce of the Free and Hanseatic City of Hamburg, health insurance companies, as well as affected persons and associations of relatives. The aim of the project, which was funded by the Federal Ministry of Education and Research (BMBF) from 2011 to 2014, was to develop and evaluate pioneering care models. In 11 scientifically accompanied subprojects, *psychenet* investigated how the care of mentally ill people can be improved and which options for prevention and better management of illnesses are effective. Within the framework of the HaLT-Hamburg research project, the present manual was developed for the implementation of a brief motivational intervention for children and adolescents who consume alcohol at risk.

We would like to take this opportunity to express our sincere thanks to the many people involved. Special thanks go to all the people who made the implementation of this elaborate research project possible in the first place. These include in particular the HaLT Hamburg counsellors Klaus Wilkens, Franka Metzner, Michael Knaack, Leona Jakubowski, Martina Teske and Corinna Liesk, who were prepared to carry out their assignments at unusual working hours and conducted the bedside interviews with marked commitment, interest and professionalism. In addition, the implementation of the study would not have been possible without our evaluation team, which also visited the adolescents in the clinics early in the morning on the weekends to interview them, and which, in addition to a whole range of different tasks during the week, carried out the follow-up telephone interviews and digitised the collected data with a great deal of commitment and perseverance. At this point, we would therefore also like to express our great thanks to Sabrina Kunze-Klempert, Victoria Winter, Janina Windsor, Kristina Wille, Elisabeth Zahn, Tharanya Seeralan, Lina Dening, Katharina Kröger, Alexandra Martin and Ida Roscher.

We would also like to mention the participating clinics, without whose cooperation and support this project could not have taken place. We would therefore like to express our sincere thanks to Dr. Barbara Hogan and Dr. Ulrike Güssow (Asklepios Klinik Altona), Prof. Dr. Norbert Veelken (Asklepios Klinik Nord Heidberg), Dr. Caroline Schmitt (Helios Mariahilf Klinik Harburg), Prof. Dr. Philippe Stock (Altonaer Kinderkrankenhaus), Prof. Dr. Ania Muntau (Universitätsklinikum Hamburg-Eppendorf), Prof. Dr. Peter Höger (Katholisches Kinderkrankenhaus Wilhelmstift) and the participating hospital staff in the six hospitals for the excellent cooperation. At this point, we would also like to thank Dr. Klaus Beelmann, head of the Hamburg Medical Association, for his support of the project.

We would also like to express our special thanks to our cooperation partner, the Department of Health and Consumer Protection of the City of Hamburg (BGV), represented by Dr. Sigrun Bever, Ms. Monika Püschl, Mr. Sven Kammerahl and Mr. Dietrich Hellge-Antoni, for their constructive cooperation, without which the implementation of this research project would also not have been possible. We would also like to make special mention of and thank Ms. Katrin Lammers (Addiction Counselling Center for Children and Adolescents Kö16a) and Mr. Udo Küstner (Drug and Alcohol Outpatient Clinic for Adolescents, Young Adults and their Families at the University Medical Center Hamburg-Eppendorf) for the many practical suggestions and the good cooperation in the development of the manual, the development and implementation of the HaLT-Hamburg training and the supervisions, as well as Ms. Katrin Lammers for the tireless outreach planning for the counsellors during the study phase.

For reasons of readability, the masculine is used throughout the manual. However, both genders are always addressed equally.

We wish the readers of this manual an inspiring and helpful reading and much success in the implementation of the intervention.

Silke Diestelkamp
Hamburg, Germany

Rainer Thomasius
Hamburg, Germany

Contents

About the Authors

Silke Diestelkamp

born in 1978, studied psychology at the University of Trier and subsequently worked with young people with behavioural problems in vocational preparation measures. Since 2010, she has been a research assistant in the project "Health Network Alcohol in Adolescence—Improving Access to Treatment for Adolescents with Risky Alcohol Consumption" at the German Centre for Addiction Research in Childhood and Adolescence (DZSKJ) at the University Medical Center Hamburg-Eppendorf (UKE) and is currently writing her doctoral thesis on the topic of "Differential Effectiveness of Brief Interventions to Reduce Risky Alcohol Consumption in Adolescents".

Rainer Thomasius

born 1957, studied medicine in Hamburg. Training in psychiatry, child and adolescent psychiatry, psychotherapy, and family therapy. Habilitation in 1994. 1999–2004 Head of the Personality and Stress Disorders Unit at the Center for Psychosocial Medicine at the University Medical Center Hamburg-Eppendorf (UKE). Since 2005 Medical Director of the "German Centre for Addiction Research in Childhood and Adolescence" at the UKE and Head of the Addiction Disorders Unit, Department of Child and Adolescent Psychiatry, Psychotherapy and Psychosomatics. Leading member of the Treatment Guidelines Commission of the German Society for Addiction Research and Addiction Therapy (DG-Sucht). Chairman of the Addiction Commission of the German Society for Child and Adolescent Psychiatry, Psychosomatics and Psychotherapy (DGKJP).

Katrin Lammers

born in 1979, studied social work/social work at the Kiel University of Applied Sciences, has been working in addiction support since graduating in 2007 and completed further training as an integrative social therapist with a focus on addiction support in 2015. Since 2010, she has been an employee of the addiction counselling Kö16a for children, adolescents, young adults and their relatives of the Authority for Health and Consumer Protection (BGV) of the City of Hamburg. In addition to counselling in individual or family settings, she is responsible for information events for adolescents, parental work, acupuncture treatment according to the NADA protocol, public relations, staff training as well as project support and coordination of the HaLT-Hamburg team.

Udo Küstner

born in 1959, studied psychology at the Johannes Gutenberg University Mainz. After his studies, he worked in different fields of psychiatry, psychotherapy and addiction. Since 2000, he has been employed as a psychological psychotherapist and research assistant in the Drug and Alcohol Outpatient Clinic for Adolescents, Young Adults and their Families at the University Medical Center Hamburg-Eppendorf.

1 Introduction

S. Diestelkamp, R. Thomasius, *Risky Alcohol Consumption among Adolescents*,
https://doi.org/10.1007/978-3-662-68635-5_1

The HaLT-Hamburg brief intervention for children and adolescents after acute alcohol intoxication was developed within the context of a research project funded by the Federal Ministry of Education and Research (BMBF) and investigated in 2011–2014 as a sub-project of the research network psychenet—Hamburg Network for Mental Health (Härter et al., 2012) in a prospective randomised-controlled study at six Hamburg clinics with regard to its effectiveness and feasibility. Based on the guideline and interview guide for so called "bridge talks" of the alcohol prevention programme HaLT–Hart am LimiT (Villa Schöpflin, 2009) and current research findings, the following study was developed in cooperation with the Addiction Counselling Center for Children and Adolescents Kö16a (Katrin Lammers) and the Drug and Alcohol Outpatient Clinic for Children, Adolescents and their Families at the University Medical Center Hamburg-Eppendorf (Udo Küstner). An intervention was developed that is both standardized and transparent and thus evaluable and transferable to other locations, but which also leaves room for individual counseling priorities. The implementation of the empathic and appreciative therapeutic basic attitude of Motivational Interviewing (MI), as it will be described in more detail later, is thus particularly taken into account. The valuable feedback of the HaLT-Hamburg counsellors and the members of the evaluation team as well as the results of the survey of the clinic staff involved were incorporated into this manual alongside the evaluation results on the effectiveness of the intervention.

The manual is divided into a theoretical part, which contains the theoretical basis of the intervention and background information about the research project. This is followed by the practical part, in which the procedure of the intervention is described in detail. Examples of conversations, explanations of the rationale of the procedure and suggestions for dealing with difficult situations are given. The manual also contains various "memo cards" which are used as a structuring aid during the intervention. The manual concludes with an appendix containing all the materials needed to carry out the intervention.

This manual is aimed at social pedagogues, psychologists, pedagogues, educationalists and medical doctors who work with children and adolescents with risky alcohol consumption. In particular, it is aimed at professionals who want to conduct a brief motivational intervention with children and adolescents after acute alcohol intoxication.

Theoretical Background

Contents

S. Diestelkamp, R. Thomasius, *Risky Alcohol Consumption among Adolescents*,
https://doi.org/10.1007/978-3-662-68635-5_2

In the following chapter, relevant background information on alcohol consumption in adolescence is presented as well as the theoretical assumptions and the conceptualisation of Motivational Interviewing.

2.1 Risky Alcohol Consumption Among Adolescents

2.1.1 Consumption and Distribution

The nationwide trend of regular alcohol consumption among 12- to 25-year-old adolescents has been declining since the 1970s (Orth & Töppich, 2015). Even among underage 12- to 17-year-olds, the proportion of adolescents who consume alcohol regularly, i.e. at least once a week, has tended to fall since data collection by the Federal Centre for Health Education began in 1979 (ibid.; ◘ Fig. 2.1).

The age of first alcohol consumption and the age of first alcohol intoxication have increased nationwide by almost 7 months since 2004 until 2014. Nevertheless, there is a stable percentage of adolescents who consume episodically to excess (Orth & Töppich, 2015). Episodic excessive consumption is often understood as binge drinking, i.e. the consumption of 5 (4 for girls) or more standard glasses of alcohol at one drinking occasion (Herring et al., 2008).

> Binge drinking is defined as the consumption of five standard alcoholic beverages at a drinking occasion for men and four standard alcoholic beverages for women.

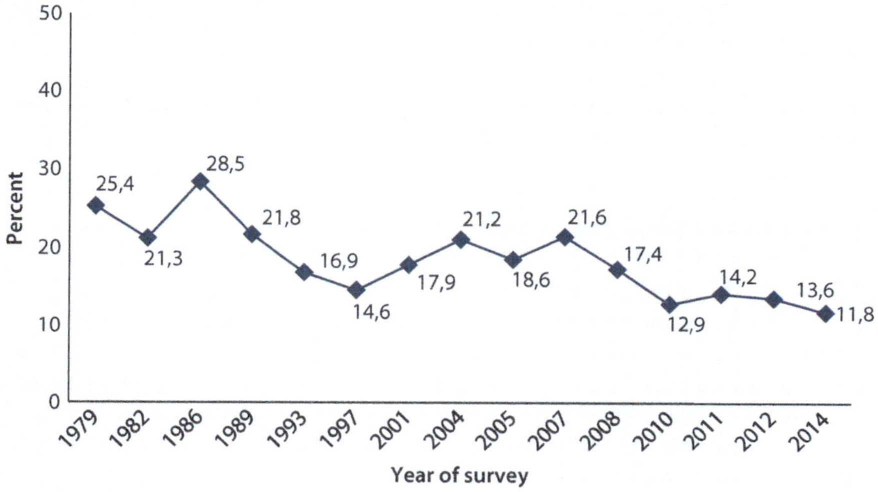

◘ **Fig. 2.1** Proportions of 12- to 17-year-olds who consume alcohol at least once a week nationwide (Orth & Töppich, 2015)

2

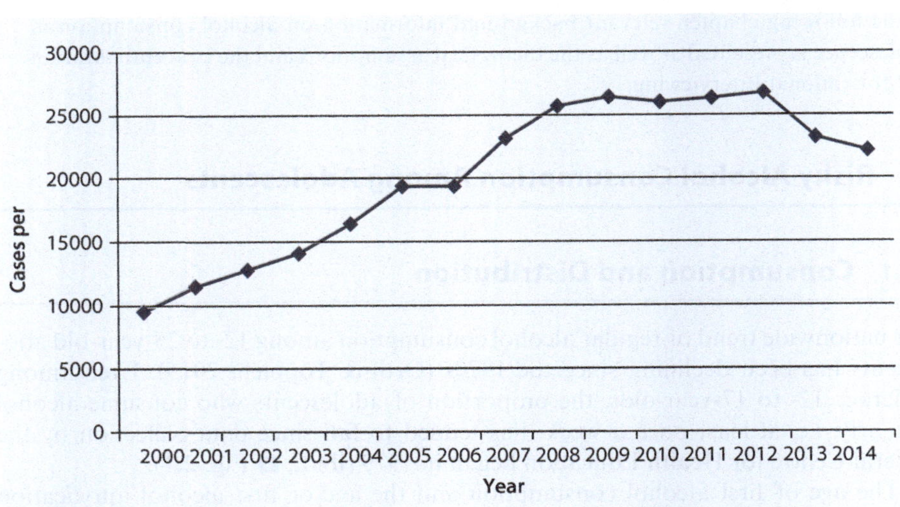

Fig. 2.2 Development of the number of inpatients under 20 years of age diagnosed with "alcohol intoxication" in hospitals nationwide (Gesundheitsberichterstattung des Bundes, 2016)

The number of adolescents up to the age of 20 years who received inpatient treatment for acute alcohol intoxication (AAI) in Germany increased from 9500 in 2000 to 22,250 in 2014, an increase of 136% (Gesundheitsberichterstattung des Bundes, 2016; Fig. 2.2). Increasing prevalence rates of adolescents requiring emergency medical treatment for acute alcohol intoxication (diagnosis F10.0, ICD 10) have been reported from various European countries in recent years (Healey et al., 2004; Fandler et al., 2008; Caflisch & Uldry, 2013; Van Hoof et al., 2010; Bitunjac & Saraga, 2009; Loukova, 2011; Kuzelová et al., 2009).

> The number of under-20s with acute alcohol intoxication has risen from about 9500 to about 22,000 cases annually since 2000.

2.1.2 Minors with Acute Alcohol Intoxication

It is likely that this increase in treatment numbers is also partly due to an increase in awareness among the population, which is expressed in the fact that an ambulance is requested even for less severely intoxicated adolescents. A study on this by Wurdak et al. (2013) found that in a community with particularly high inpatient treatment rates for minors with AAI, the average blood alcohol concentration of treated adolescents was lower and the willingness of the population to request an ambulance was higher than in a comparison community with lower treatment rates. Nevertheless, it should be noted that among minors requiring emergency medical treatment for alcohol intoxication, there is a higher proportion of children and adolescents who are risky substance users and exposed to further developmental hazards compared to the general population. For example, higher prevalences of alcohol abuse, alcohol dependence, binge drinking, tobacco use, and illicit substance use have been observed among children and adolescents with AAI than in the general population (Groß et al., 2016a). In the HaLT Hamburg sample, a very high proportion (63.6%) of children and adolescents were observed to receive a positive screening result for risky alcohol use (Wartberg et al., n.d.). A study in Bavaria found that minors with AAI drank less frequently than adolescents in the general population (2.8 vs. 5.0 days in the past 30 days), but consumed larger amounts when they did drink (36.4 g vs. 22.3 g of pure alcohol per drinking day; Kraus et al., 2013). Drinking pattern analyses showed that 21.5% of minors with AAI can be classified as habitually risky alcohol consumers and 16.5% as habitually high-risk consumers (Diestelkamp et al., 2015).

In addition, psychosocial distress was also found to be higher in this target group than in the general population. Adolescents who have received emergency medical treatment with an AAI have a sixfold increased risk of being affected by severe developmental vulnerabilities, such as family violence, school problems, delinquency, and perpetration and victimization of violence (Kuttler et al., 2016). By their mid-twenties, young adults hospitalized as minors with an AAI have significantly higher prevalence of a serious alcohol-related disorder (8% vs. 1% in a comparison sample without an AAI), are more likely to use illicit substances (20% vs. 10%), and are more likely to report delinquent behavior (50% vs. 35%; Groß et al., 2016b).

> Alcohol intoxication of a minor does not necessarily mean that he or she habitually consumes alcohol in a risky manner and is psychosocially severely burdened. However, the proportion of at-risk adolescents in this target group is higher than in comparable age groups in the general population.

2.2 Risks and Consequences

Alcohol use is one of the three most significant risk factors contributing to the global burden of disease (Lim et al., 2012). For children and adolescents with episodic excessive alcohol consumption,[1] the immediate and medium-term consequences of risky alcohol consumption in particular pose a major threat (Stolle et al., 2009). Adolescents who consume risky amounts of alcohol have an increased risk of experiencing violent acts, both as perpetrators and victims (Swahn et al., 2004). In addition to psychological consequences such as trauma, injuries and conflicts with police are common consequences of alcohol-related violence. In an alcoholized state, other risky behaviors, such as drunk driving, also occur more frequently (Sindelar et al., 2004). Furthermore, in conjunction with depressive disorders and critical life events, episodic excessive drinking increases the risk of suicide attempts in adolescents. If adolescents lose consciousness due to excessive drinking, severe somatic complications may result from hypothermia or aspiration of vomit. Furthermore, for girls in particular, unwanted and/or unprotected sexual contact while intoxicated poses a risk that can lead to unintended pregnancies and STIs, and even trauma from rape experiences (Champion et al., 2004). Girls who engage in binge drinking have a threefold increased risk of becoming victims of unwanted sexual acts (Champion

---

1 The terms "episodic excessive drinking", "binge drinking" and "binge drinking" are used synonymously here. Herring et al. (2008), for example, point out the blurred terminology.

et al., 2004). Early and frequent episodic excessive drinking is associated with an increased risk for later development of a substance-related disorder (Viner & Taylor, 2007). The risk of developing an alcohol-related disorder (harmful use or dependence syndrome) increases with a younger age of onset of frequent excessive drinking (Stolle et al., 2009). The risk of using other (illegal) psychotropic substances also increases.

Despite the generally decreasing trend in underage drinking, there are children and adolescents who consume excessively and are thus exposed to a variety of acute, medium and long-term risks and impairments.

2.3 Consumption Motives and Consumer Expectations

The motives for excessive alcohol consumption among adolescents are manifold. According to Silbereisen and Reese (2001), alcohol consumption and excessive drinking can also take on functions in coping with developmental tasks in adolescence. Thus, episodic binge drinking can be an expression of social protest and represent an intentional violation of norms. It can fulfil the function of individuation from parents or express membership of a particular peer group (Table 2.1).

Excessive alcohol consumption can also be a consequence of inexperience and ignorance or serve as a coping strategy for stress, anxiety or other emotional problems. Last but not least, the disinhibiting effect of alcohol is often a motive for consumption, since, for example, it makes it easier to establish contact and initiate

Table 2.1 Functions of substance use according to Silbereisen and Reese (2001)

Development tasks	Functions of substance use
- Know who you are and what you want (Self Concept and Identity)	- Expression of personal style - Search for cross-border, mind-expanding experiences and experiences
- Building friendships; establishing intimate relationships	- Facilitating access to peer groups - Excessive ritualized behavior - Contacting opposite-sex peers
- Breaking away from one's parents	- Demonstrate independence from parents - Deliberate violation of parental control
- Adoption of adult behaviours	- Demonstration, anticipation of adulthood
- Life design, planning	- Participation in subcultural lifestyle - Have fun and enjoy
- Own value system	- Intentional violation of the norm - Expression of social protest
- Developmental problems	- Substitute goal of denied normative development goals - Stress and emotion management (emergency response)

romantic relationships. These social motives are most frequently cited by adolescents as reasons for consuming alcohol, significantly more frequently than enhancing positive affect ("drinking to enhance"; Cooper et al., 1995) or avoiding negative affect ("drinking to cope"; Cooper et al., 1995; Kuntsche et al., 2005).

> Alcohol consumption in adolescence can have functions in coping with developmental tasks, e.g. with regard to identity development and peer group affiliation.

While motives for consumption reflect the reasons for consumption, i.e. the intention to bring about a certain desired outcome (Cox & Klinger, 1988), efficacy expectations reflect personal beliefs regarding positive or negative (i.e. intended and unintended) effects of consumption (Kuntsche et al., 2005). Alcohol efficacy expectations influence the age of initiation into alcohol use (Jester et al., 2015), use itself, and the effectiveness of alcohol interventions (Black et al., 2012).

In a representative survey among school students in Germany aged 15–16 years, two thirds of the adolescents stated "having fun" as the most frequently expected effect of alcohol consumption (Hibell et al., 2012; ▫ Table 2.2). Only about one third of the adolescents expected their health to be endangered by alcohol consumption, and only one quarter of the respondents stated that they were concerned that they might do things under the influence of alcohol that they might regret later.

> The majority of adolescents consume alcohol for social motives and have a low perception of potential negative consequences of consumption.

▫ Table 2.2 Alcohol effect expectations of 15- to 16-year-olds in selected German states (data in percent) (Hibell et al., 2012)

	Total	Boys	Girls
Have a lot of fun	76	77	75
Feel more sociable	65	64	66
Feel relaxed	55	63	49
Feel happy	55	57	53
Forget my problems	48	49	47
Endangering my health	37	36	38
Do things I regret later	25	25	25
Getting a hangover	28	27	28
Can't stop drinking	12	11	12
Problems with the police	10	13	7
Feeling sick	11	11	11

2.4 Models of Adolescent Alcohol Consumption

The consumption of alcohol in adolescence fulfils significantly different functions than in adulthood and is always to be understood in preventive work against this youth-specific background. Alcohol consumption in adolescence is therefore often conceptualised as risky behaviour (Jessor, 1987, 1991; Wiers et al., 2007, 2010; Gibbons et al., 2003); in contrast, models of abuse and dependence in adulthood (see West, 2013, for an overview) often understand alcohol abuse as a dysfunctional coping strategy (e.g. Orford, 2001).

In the following, three models with direct application to the development and maintenance of adolescent alcohol consumption are presented, each with a different relevant focus.

1. The *Motivational Model of Alcohol Use* (Cox & Klinger, 1988, 2004, 2011) with a particular focus on the role of motivation,
2. the *Social Reaction Model of Adolescent Health Risk* (Gibbons et al., 2003), which places a special focus on the youth-specific social embeddedness of alcohol consumption and thus on the significance of consumption for identity development as a central developmental task in adolescence,
3. The *Dual Process Model of Adolescent Risk Taking* (Wiers et al., 2007, 2010), which highlights the dialectic of reflective, controlled and automatic, impulsive processes in the emergence and maintenance of risky alcohol use in adolescence.

2.4.1 Motivational Model of Alcohol Use

This biopsychosocial model (Cox & Klinger, 1988, 2004, 2011) was not specifically designed for adolescent drinking, but provides a very good overview of the influencing factors and motivational processes involved in the decision to drink or abstain from alcohol. In line with recent dual-process models (see Wiers et al., 2007, 2010), this model also assumes that both conscious and unconscious factors influence the drinking decision. Here, previous experiences with alcohol consumption as well as current drinking circumstances affect the perceived benefits of a positive drinking decision. Previous experiences are understood to be personality traits, biological predispositions as well as sociocultural and environmental factors. Depending on the extent of these individual factors, alcohol consumption has been reinforced to varying degrees by previous experiences and thus influences learned cognitive and conditioned reactions to the consumption of alcohol. According to this model, the central factor is the incentive value of alcohol consumption, which is dependent on the expected reduction of negative affect or the reinforcement of positive affect, or both. In adolescents, as described in ► Sect. 2.3, the reinforcement of positive affect is expected to be a much more frequent drinking motive than in adults. Another key element of the model is the comparison of the expected affective benefits of alcohol consumption with the affective benefits of alternative sources of reward. A weighing of these expected consequences of the behaviour, influenced by cognitive variables such as values and beliefs, then leads, according to the model, to the decision to drink or not to drink (◘ Fig. 2.3). This model illustrates how motivation to drink or not to drink can arise and therefore provides a basis for deriving an intervention strategy. In

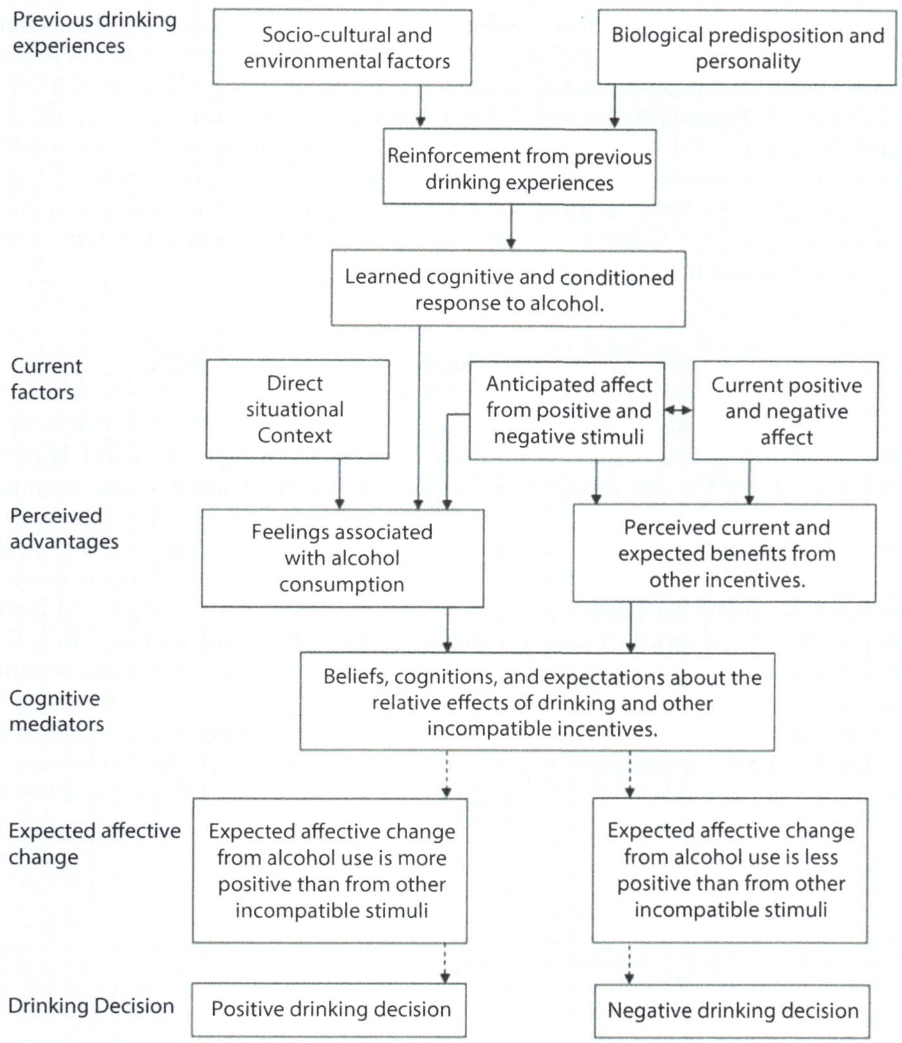

Fig. 2.3 The Motivational Model of Alcohol Use. (Cox & Klinger, 2011, courtesy of John Wiley & Sons)

particular, this model highlights the importance of efficacy expectations and alternative sources of reward, two elements that offer promising approaches for intervention.

Thus, this model belongs to the widely used expectancy-value theories, which also include the influential theories of health behavior Theory of Reasoned Action (Fishbein & Ajzen, 1975) and its extension in the Theory of Planned Behavior (Ajzen, 1985, 1991). These models basically assume that a behavioral intention always precedes the corresponding behavior. A behavioral intention is the result of a deliberation process involving attitudes regarding the behavior and the expected consequences of a behavior, as well as perceived subjective and social norms regarding that behavior. When such behavioral plans are matched with appropriate opportunities to perform the behavior and resources to implement them, behavioral goals can be achieved. The Theory of Planned Behavior has been widely tested in its utility for predicting health behaviors and has high predictive value (Armitage & Conner, 2001). Nevertheless, the model has weaknesses, particularly in predicting impulsive and irrational behaviors, such as adolescent risk-taking behavior. Gibbons et al. (2003) therefore developed a model for predicting adolescent risk behavior based on the Theory of Planned Behavior.

2.4.2 Social Reaction Model of Adolescent Health Risk

The importance of the social embeddedness of adolescent alcohol consumption is particularly emphasised in the Social Reaction Model of Adolescent Health Risk by Gibbons et al. (2003). According to this model, alcohol use in adolescence is understood as a social action and, unlike in adulthood, is conceptualized primarily as a form of risk behavior. Gibbons and colleagues hypothesize that two distinct pathways lead to adolescent risk behaviors: First, a conscious and deliberative process in which, according to the Theory of Planned Behavior, a conscious behavioral intention precedes the behavior. A second pathway, on the other hand, describes how risk behaviour emerges without conscious intention and often as a reaction to found social situations (◘ Fig. 2.4).

The central assumption of the model is therefore that risk behaviour in adolescence is often a reaction to social situations that "entices" such behaviour. The second assumption of the model concerns the context and function of adolescent risk behav-

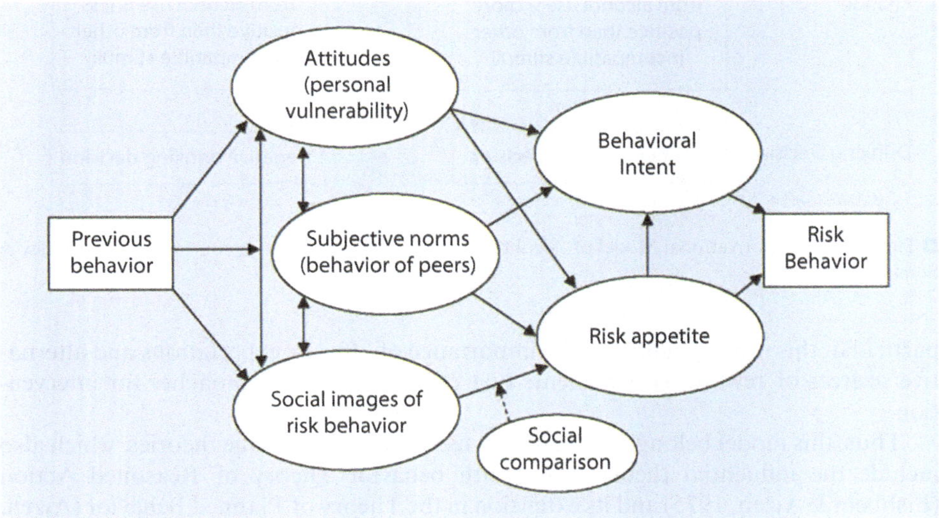

◘ **Fig. 2.4** The Social Reaction Model of Adolescent Health Risk. (Gibbons et al., 2003, courtesy of John Wiley & Sons)

iour. As described in ► Sect. 2.3, alcohol use in adolescence may serve functions in achieving various developmental tasks, particularly functions related to identity development, the central developmental task in adolescence (Havighurst, 1948). The model assumes that certain social images are associated with the consumption of alcohol or other substances in adolescence. In a third assumption, it is formulated that these social images, the so-called prototypes, lead to a social comparison process in which the adolescent compares himself with the prototypes and, in the case of a positive evaluation, strives to integrate this social image into his own identity perception. A number of studies have been able to show that the perceived social prototypes have a significant influence on the exercise of risk behaviour in adolescence (e.g. consumption of alcohol or tobacco; Chassin et al., 1981, 1985; Burton et al., 1989).

Another central construct of this model is behavioral willingness, which describes openness to risk behavior. This construct takes into account the fact that adolescents often state that they do not intend to engage in risky behavior. However, when a risk situation occurs unintentionally, there is often willingness to perform the corresponding risk behavior or there is no motivation not to perform the risk behavior. Adolescents with a high risk propensity in the sense of the model are exposed to a particular risk because they do not prepare themselves for the risk behaviour (e.g. in the case of excessive alcohol consumption they do not organise the way home in advance).

In this sense, the Social Reaction Model also assumes two processes that together influence adolescent risk behavior: a deliberative, rational process and a less intentional process that reacts to external influences. With this assumption, the model reflects the assumptions of current dual-process models (Strack & Deutsch, 2004; Wiers et al., 2007), which also assume, based on neurobiological research, that behavior is influenced by two processes, a reflective, conscious process and an automatic, impulsive process. These models differ from the Social Reaction Model primarily in their assumption of different factors that influence the situation-specific influence of the two processes. In the following, the Dual Process Model of Adolescent Risk Taking by Wiers et al. (2007, 2010) is presented.

2.4.3 The Dual Process Model of Adolescent Risk Behaviour

The dual process model of adolescent risk behaviour according to Wiers et al. (2007, 2010) assumes, as described above, that adolescent risk behaviour, such as excessive alcohol consumption, is influenced by two processes. One is a reflective, controlled process and the other is an impulsive process. Similar to Cox and Klinger (2011) and Gibbons et al. (2003), Wiers et al. (2010) hypothesize that past experiences, context, situation, and emotional and cognitive factors have an influence on risk behaviors. In contrast to the previous models, Wiers and co-workers emphasise from their neurobiological perspective the importance of the ability and motivation to exercise self-control as a reflective process, as well as the importance of automatic affective associations and 'approach-avoidance' tendencies in the development of risk behaviours (◘ Fig. 2.5). The capacity for self-control varies interindividually, is subject to a developmental maturation process (Steinberg, 2010), and is influenced by environmental factors. For example, acute alcohol consumption reduces cognitive processing

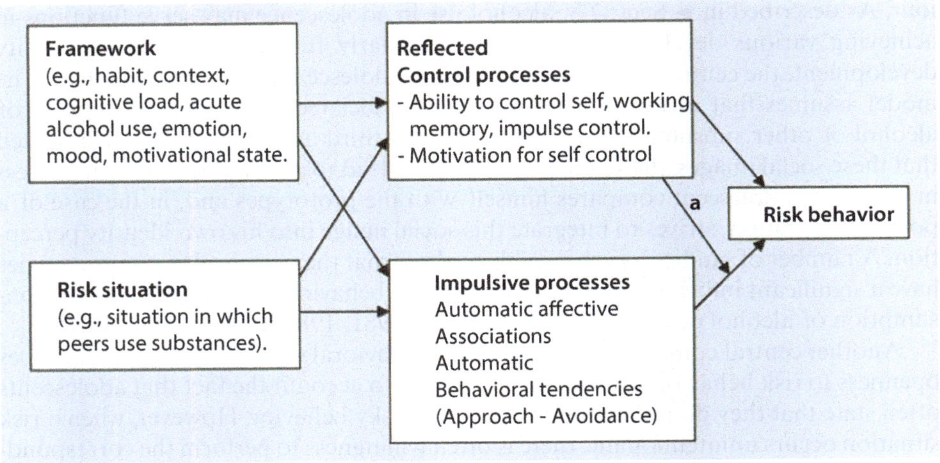

Fig. 2.5 The dual process model of adolescent risk behaviour (abridged). (After Wiers et al., 2010, © 2010 Wiers, Ames, Hofmann, Krank and Stacy)

capacity ("ego depletion"; Baumeister & Vohs, 2007) and can thus lead to a reduced ability and motivation for self-control, resulting in a strengthening of impulsive processes. Similarly, habit, cognitive load, emotion, mood, and motivational state can affect both reflective and impulsive processes. Impulsive processes are primarily understood in this model as automatic behavioral tendencies, i.e., an unconscious behavioral disposition to respond to a stimulus (e.g., alcohol) with approach or avoidance.

For practical work with young people who consume alcohol at risk, the effects of acute alcohol consumption on risk behaviour (e.g. further alcohol consumption or other risk behaviours), as well as the influence of impulsive processes on risk behaviour, are of particular importance. The moderating effect of reflective processes on the influence of impulsive processes (Fig. 2.5, arrow a) formulated in the model is also an important starting point for preventive work.

2.5 Risk and Protective Factors for Later Harm from Alcohol Consumption

Minors who consume alcohol at risk are exposed to a high risk of experiencing one or more of the acute consequences of risky consumption, some of which can be severe. A proportion of these young people are also at risk of developing an alcohol-related disorder in adulthood. In a study of 277 young adults surveyed 5–13 years after treatment for alcohol intoxication, 12.6% met DSM-IV criteria for alcohol abuse and 19.9% met criteria for alcohol dependence, a significantly higher percentage than in the general population (Groß et al., 2016a). Predictors of later binge drinking, alcohol dependence, and lower life satisfaction were identified as male gender, use of illicit substances in adolescence, and behavioral problems associated with externalizing disorders, such as running away and truancy. In addition to delinquency and poor academic performance, a recent longitudinal study of 746 adolescents in

Canada found that parental monitoring and peer substance use also had a significant impact on the course of alcohol use in childhood and adolescence (Yamada et al., 2016). In this study, externalising behavioural problems were also identified as predictors of particularly severe courses.

Many adolescents reduce their consumption with the transition into young adulthood ("maturing out"; Lee et al., 2013). For those who do not "grow out" of harmful use on their own, one or more intra- or inter-individual risk factors are often present. According to a review by Jordan and Sack (2009), these include:

- genetic predisposition,
- low socioeconomic status of the family of origin,
- gender of the adolescent "male",
- problematic alcohol consumption by other family members (especially parents),
- childhood neglect and abuse,
- early school failure,
- Aggressiveness,
- affiliation with alcohol-using peer group in late childhood and adolescence,
- externalizing behavior disorders (social behavior disorder, untreated ADHD),
- Delinquency in early adolescence,
- impulsivity and curiosity ("sensation/novelty seeking") in adolescence.

Jordan and Sack (2009) identified protective factors for later harm from alcohol use:

- balanced temper,
- social and emotional skills,
- few conflicts with parents,
- positive parent-child communication,
- religiosity/spirituality in adolescence.

In the work with children and adolescents who consume alcohol at risk, it is therefore always a question of recognising risk factors as indicators of possible danger and strengthening protective factors as possible resources for the prevention of later damage caused by alcohol consumption.

2.6 Recognition of Risky Alcohol Consumption

The distinction between "normative" experimental consumption and harmful alcohol consumption is often difficult in adolescence, especially for parents. A manifest alcohol dependence according to the criteria of the ICD-10 is rather rarely observed in adolescence.

Criteria for the Dependence Syndrome According to ICD-10 (Dilling & Freyberger, 2001)

Three or more of the following criteria must have been met simultaneously within the last year:

1. A strong desire or some kind of compulsion to consume substances or alcohol.
2. Decreased ability to control the onset, cessation, and amount of substance use.

3. A physical withdrawal syndrome
4. Evidence of tolerance
5. Progressive neglect of other interests in favour of substance use
6. Continued substance use despite evidence of clear harmful consequences

Criteria for Harmful Use According to ICD-10 (Dilling & Freyberger, 2001)

For the diagnosis, all of the following criteria must apply:

1. The diagnosis requires actual damage to physical or mental health.
2. Harmful consumer behaviour is often criticised by others and has various negative social consequences.
3. Harmful use is not diagnosable in dependence syndrome, psychotic disorder, or other substance-related disorders

In addition, consumption in adolescence often has different effects than in adulthood, which is why the application of the ICD-10 criteria should be limited. For example, significant harmful effects of alcohol consumption on social relationships, school performance and coping with everyday life are often observed without the criteria of tolerance development or physical withdrawal syndrome being fulfilled. Newcomb and Bentler (1989) therefore formulated criteria for distinguishing experimental ("normative") alcohol consumption from alcohol abuse in childhood and adolescence, which allow a more holistic view of the effects of consumption on adolescent development:

Criteria for Distinguishing Experimental Alcohol Use from Alcohol Abuse in Childhood and Adolescence (Newcomb & Bentler, 1989)

- Consumption circumstances

  Indications of alcohol abuse are given if excessive consumption takes place over a longer period of time or if the alcohol consumption occurs in inappropriate situations (e.g. school). Thus, both the amount and duration of consumption as well as the circumstances of consumption are taken into account.
- Person

  If the adolescent's age-appropriate development is jeopardized by alcohol consumption, or if the adolescent is developmentally unable to adequately assess the risk posed by alcohol consumption, alcohol abuse is suspected.
- Reaction

  Impairments in coping with everyday life, withdrawal symptoms and other signs of physical dependence indicate abuse.
- Consequences

  Signs of abuse include impairment of social relationships, health and the occurrence of unlawful acts related to alcohol consumption.

To support the detection of risky alcohol consumption, the use of short screening tests is recommended. In the introductory interview of the HaLT-Hamburg intervention, the screening test CRAFFT-d (Tossmann et al., 2009) is used as standard, which has proven to be a valid instrument for detecting risky consumption (Wartberg et al., 2016; ► Fig. 5.2). If an adolescent answers two or more questions with yes, there is a reasonable suspicion of risky alcohol consumption.

For people with risky alcohol consumption, the implementation of brief motivational interventions is recommended. In the AWMF-S3 treatment guideline for screening, diagnosis and treatment of alcohol-related disorders in childhood and adolescence (Thomasius et al., 2016), the use is also recommended for children and adolescents. Brief motivational interventions are particularly suitable as an early intervention to trigger and strengthen intrinsic motivation for further treatment and/or independent reduction of risky consumption patterns. Due to their brevity (between 10 and 60 min, one to three sessions), they are particularly suitable for implementation in settings where possibly only few contacts or only one contact with the client is feasible.

2.7 Effectiveness of Brief Motivational Interventions

The effectiveness of alcohol-specific brief interventions in primary care has been investigated in a large number of randomised-controlled trials and is now considered well established (Kaner et al., 2007; Nilsen et al., 2008; Schmidt et al., 2016). However, significantly fewer studies are available for adolescents and young adults. The largest number of randomized-controlled trials (RCTs) have been conducted with American college students. In a meta-analysis of randomised-controlled intervention trials on the effectiveness of brief interventions for binge drinking, effect sizes of $d = 0.20$ (small effect) were found in this target group at different follow-up time points (Carey et al., 2007); according to the authors, these are "typical" in the addiction field. In the case of non-motivated adolescents who were "prescribed" participation in a brief intervention as a condition (e.g. by the campus police, which is widespread in the USA), the brief motivational intervention proved to be superior to a standard intervention, especially with two booster sessions.

The emergency room setting seems to be suitable in principle for brief interventions with the target group of adolescents (Monti et al., 1999). In particular, four RCTs by a US research group were able to report effects of brief motivational interventions for adolescents and young adults treated in emergency departments due to an alcohol-related incident on various outcomes (Monti et al., 1999, 2007; Spirito et al., 2004, 2011). Some improvements remained stable over 12 months (such as reduced number of binge drinking events and mean blood alcohol concentration); however, some outcome variables remained unaffected (such as alcohol-associated injuries and drunk driving). In Germany, the effectiveness of a brief motivational intervention for adolescents and young adults under 21 years of age after AAI was investigated in a Hamburg pilot study (Stolle et al., 2013). Study participants reported a significant reduction in drinking in the last 30 days 6 months after the intervention. This result should be taken as an indication of the effectiveness of the intervention, but it should be noted that due to the lack of comparison to drinking behaviour in a control group, no causal statements could be made about the causes of the reduction in consumption. Reis et al. (2009) investigated the effects of implementing a brief motivational intervention and community alcohol prevention strategies (project HaLT–Hart am LimiT) on the 12-month prevalences of minors with AAI in two comparison regions. They found a 20% decrease in AAI prevalence in the experimental region and a 33% increase in prevalence in the control region. This study thus also provided data supporting the effectiveness of this approach. Another study in Germany also found that minors with AAI who received a brief motivational intervention in the clinic had significantly reduced both their frequency of drinking and binge drinking 1 month after the clinic stay (Wurdak et al., 2016). Again, however, this study was unable to compare trends in drinking behaviour with a control group who had received no intervention. What was tested was whether the use of a tablet-based intervention module on drinking motives was associated with greater reductions in alcohol consumption than the stand-alone intervention. It was found that girls benefited from the additional element, whereas boys did not.

Overall, there are few randomised-controlled trials of the effectiveness of brief interventions for adolescents in the emergency setting who are being treated for their alcohol use (Yuma-Guerrero et al., 2012). In their systematic review, Newton et al. (2013) analysed a subset of studies examining the effectiveness of 'targeted' brief interventions for adolescents in the emergency setting, i.e. brief interventions aimed at adolescents being treated for their alcohol use. They conclude that the small number of randomised-controlled trials and the heterogeneity of effects do not allow a conclusive assessment of effectiveness for this target group given the current state of studies. A systematic review on the effectiveness of brief motivational interventions for adolescents in emergency settings who are being treated for their alcohol consumption, which was conducted within the framework of the HaLT Hamburg study, was able to include a total of 7 randomised-controlled studies, 6 practice projects, one non-randomised pilot study and one observational study due to extended search criteria (Diestelkamp et al., 2016). Due to the heterogeneity of the study designs and the reported effects, this review also concludes that the effectiveness of alcohol-related brief interventions for this target group cannot currently be conclusively assessed. However, the high number of published practice projects reflects the need for effective interventions in clinical practice. Brief motivational interventions are based on the interviewing approach of Motivational Interviewing (MI) according to Miller and Rollnick (2002, 2013), which is presented in the following.

2.8 Motivational Interviewing According to Miller and Rollnick

Motivational interviewing (MI) is a method described by Miller and Rollnick (2002, 2013), which has become increasingly popular in the counselling of people with addiction problems. In contrast to earlier concepts of addiction and dependence, according to which people must first have reached a low point before a change in behaviour can be brought about, Miller and Rollnick assume that it is precisely early intervention that is promising.

The HaLT Hamburg intervention was originally developed on the basis of the conceptualisation of MI from 2002 (Miller & Rollnick, 2002). The content and procedure of the brief intervention are described in the practical part of the manual as they were originally elaborated and evaluated in the associated study (▶ Chap. 3). New recommendations for the implementation of the intervention, as derived from the 2013 third edition of Miller and Rollnick's standard work, are referenced in appropriate footnotes. In the following theory section of the manual, the more differentiated elaboration of the theoretical assumptions of MI according to Miller and Rollnick (2013) is presented.

Motivational interviewing is based on the assumption that in most cases people are ambivalent about potentially harmful behaviours. That is, tendencies to give up a certain risky behaviour are opposed by tendencies to repeat or maintain this behaviour. Counseling practice has shown that confrontation and compelling argumentation to abandon a risk behavior often have the opposite effect. People, and especially adolescents, often argue for the position *not* taken by their counterpart in a conversation. If the counsellor argues that the adolescent urgently needs to limit his alcohol consumption, it is very likely that the adolescent will take the opposite position and present a series of arguments proving that his consumption is unproblematic in his eyes.

This example illustrates another important basic assumption in MI. In MI, the counsellor does not see himself as an expert who passes on his knowledge of relevant risk behaviour to the client. Rather, MI is about the counsellor trying to get to know the client's point of view as comprehensively as possible. This requires a respectful and appreciative attitude on the part of the counsellor. A young person who feels that his behaviour and motives are disapproved of and criticised will not open up and trustingly explain his world view and especially possible doubts about it.

In this context, Miller and Rollnick refer to the so-called corrective reflex (Miller & Rollnick, 2013). Professionals in the helping professions are often confronted with individuals who engage in harmful behaviour, such as excessive alcohol consumption, with serious negative consequences for themselves and their environment. Looking at the serious negative consequences, such as damage to health or, in the case of adolescent drinking, the acute dangers associated with binge drinking due to loss of control or acts of violence, often leads helpers to feel the need to "open the eyes" of the client so that he or she finally takes the decisive steps to change the risky behaviour.

However, this understandable and good intention to motivate the client to change behaviour by illustrating the negative consequences of the status quo often turns out to be counterproductive in practice. In such a situation, the counsellor acts as a proponent of change and thus provokes the client to take the opposite position and put forward arguments in favour of maintaining the status quo. The goal of MI is therefore not to give in to the corrective reflex, but rather to frame a conversation in such a way that the client explores his or her own values and goals, thereby becoming aware of possible discrepancies with current behavior and thus creating intrinsic motivation to change behavior. The counsellor accompanies and supports this process with the aim that the client becomes an advocate for his or her own change. In this sense, MI is a directive type of interviewing because, unlike early client-centered approaches to interviewing, it has an explicit goal of changing harmful behaviors.

Ambivalence is understood as a normal phase of behavioural change and the confrontation with it is at the centre of the counselling interview. Motivation to change is by no means a prerequisite, but rather the goal of successful counselling (Demmel, 2003).

The MI has been continuously developed since its first description by Stephen Miller in 1983. It is now used in a wide variety of settings (GP practices, clinics, counselling centres) and for a wide variety of target groups (diabetes patients, pregnant women, HIV-infected people). In addition, the effectiveness and mechanisms of action of MI have been investigated in a large number of studies, the results of which have constantly stimulated the further development of the theoretical basis of MI. In the most recent edition of the textbook *Motivational Interviewing* (Miller & Rollnick, 2013), three definitions of MI are given, each with different objectives. In the German edition, the definitions are translated as follows:

Definitions for Motivational Interviewing (After Miller & Rollnick, 2015, p. 473)

General definition:

A collaborative style of conversation aimed at strengthening a person's self-motivation and self-commitment to change.

Therapeutic definition:

A person-centered style of counseling that addresses the common problem of ambivalence about an impending change.

Technical Definition:

A collaborative, goal-oriented style of communication in which special attention is given to talking about change. It is designed to strengthen a person's motivation and self-commitment to achieving a particular goal by elaborating and exploring, in an atmosphere of acceptance and compassion, the person's own reasons for which change would be good for them.

2.8.1 The Basic Therapeutic Attitude in MI

The special characteristic of MI, the basic therapeutic attitude, is at the heart of this counselling approach and has remained practically unchanged since its first conceptualisation. This basic attitude is more than just an attitude to be adopted in a therapeutic conversation. It is an expression of an image of humanity based on the fact that every person has a right to respect and dignity. This means that the client's point of view is always respected and not questioned as the basis of the conversation. Accordingly, each person possesses wisdom about themselves and the greatest expert knowledge about themselves. In recognition of this, the counsellor always respects the client's autonomy. It is solely within the client's power to change his or her behavior or not to do so. Change imposed from the outside cannot be sustainable in the understanding of MI. Accordingly, the therapeutic relationship is one of partnership in which there is no power imbalance between the instructor and the instructed. Miller and Rollnick (2013) use the image of counsellor and client sitting side by side on the sofa, leafing through the photo album of the client's life together. Such a shared, partnership perspective on risk behaviors should be taken in MI.

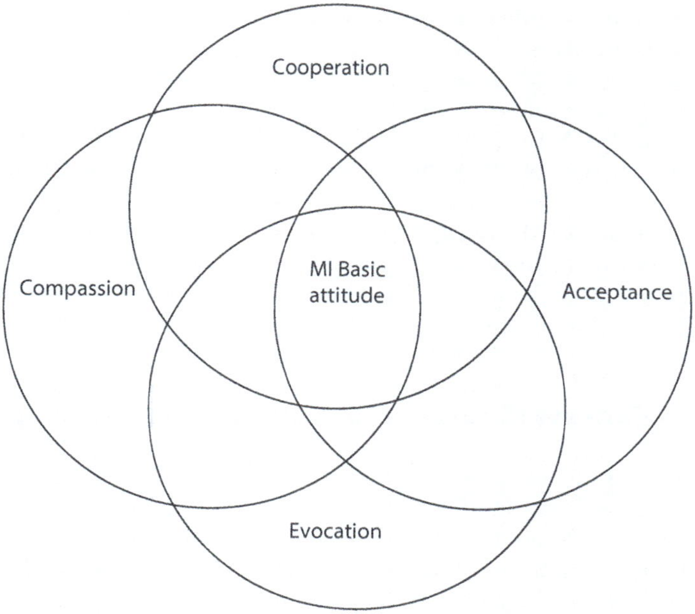

Fig. 2.6 The four core aspects of the therapeutic stance in MI. (From Miller & Rollnick, 2015, with kind permission of Lambertus)

The four core aspects of the MI basic attitude (Fig. 2.6) are

1. Partnership/Cooperation,
2. Acceptance,
3. Compassion and
4. Evocation.

The accepting basic attitude finds its implementation in four areas. First, in the recognition and support of the client's autonomy. Secondly, in the exercise of "precise empathy". This is understood to mean empathizing with the client's point of view as precisely and non-judgmentally as possible. By specifying "precise", Miller and Rollnick point out that MI is not just about creating an empathic atmosphere in the conversation. Rather, it is about an attitude that involves a genuine interest in getting to know and understand the other person's lifeworld as precisely as possible, since this clarification of a shared perspective is the basis for a fruitful conversation. The interest in engaging with the young person's point of view, without judging or even criticising it, generates acceptance rather than resistance. The essential goal is to identify motives for action through open questions and reflection and to address the underlying needs. Miller and Rollnick cite the third area of the basic accepting attitude as unconditional appreciation of the client as a prerequisite for an open conversation in which the client can address perceived weaknesses or doubts without fear of criticism or condemnation. The fourth area of acceptance is appreciation, which particularly reflects the resource orientation of MI. Instead of identifying and working on deficits and problems, the counsellor in MI focuses on identifying strengths and efforts and strengthening them through appreciation.

As the third core aspect of the basic MI attitude, in addition to cooperation/partnership and acceptance, Miller and Rollnick name compassion, meaning the authentic striving of the counsellor to use MI for the benefit of the client. This aspect has the background that MI was also used in the past to influence clients' purchasing decisions in the interest of corporations with correspondingly questionable benefits for the clients.

The fourth aspect of the MI approach is evocation. Evocation is the assumption that clients have expert knowledge about themselves and therefore also solutions to their problems and that the task of the counsellor is therefore to support the client in bringing forth these solutions ("evoking").

2.8.2 The 4-Process Model of Motivational Interviewing

While Miller and Rollnick in their earlier conceptualization of MI (2002) postulated two successive phases of MI (triggering motivation, strengthening self-efficacy) and four principles, they describe four processes of MI in the current elaboration of the theoretical basis. The four processes build on each other chronologically, each subsequent process can only begin when the previous one has taken place. When a new process begins, the previous one does not end, but continues to run in parallel and in recurring loops with the added processes (◘ Fig. 2.7).

According to the 4-process model of MI, relationship building in accordance with the basic attitudes of MI (the "spirit" of MI) is a prerequisite for all other processes. Once an appreciative and cooperative relationship has been established, the next process is focusing. This process involves clarifying the goals of the conversation. Since MI has a clear objective (changing harmful behaviour), clarifying these objectives at the beginning of the conversation is essential and indispensable for the further processes. In a brief motivational intervention with an adolescent after acute alcohol intoxication, one goal for the vast majority of adolescents, regardless of their habitual use of alcohol, is to avoid another hospital stay due to their alcohol use. If an adolescent rejects this goal for him/herself, it may indicate a dissonance in the relationship between the counselor and the adolescent. How to deal with such situations is discussed in more detail in ► Sect. 2.8.4.

Once a focus on one or more goals of the conversation has been established, the process of evocation follows. This is the process in which MI stands out from other approaches. During evocation, the counsellor uses certain communication strategies

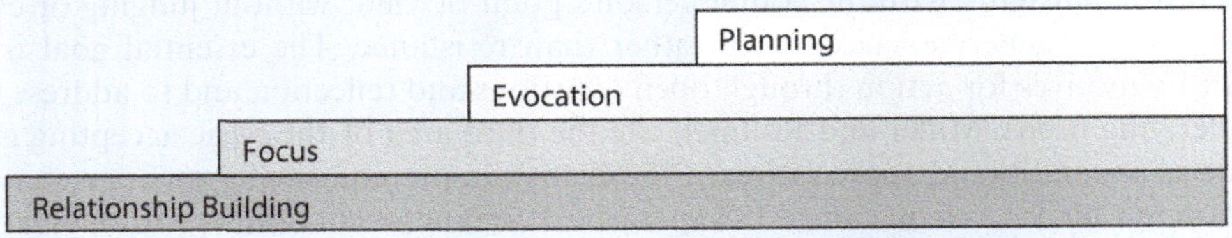

◘ **Fig. 2.7** The 4-process model of MI. (Miller & Rollnick, 2015, with kind permission of Lambertus)

to specifically trigger and reinforce statements from the client that are in favour of change ("change talk"). Change talk refers to any statements made by the adolescent that refer to a possible change in current problematic behavior. Change talk can include statements about negative aspects of the status quo as well as positive aspects of a change in behaviour. These statements by the adolescent are specifically elicited in MI through open-ended questions and reflective listening, and are especially reinforced through reflective listening. Change talk can be statements that reflect a desire for change, refer to the ability to bring about change, address reasons for change, or articulate a need or necessity for change. In English, the abbreviation DARN ("desire", "ability", "reason", "*need*") is used for this systematization of the forms of expression of change talk. In addition to these expressions of "preparatory" change talk, there are expressions of "mobilizing" change talk. These are statements that refer to the imminent implementation of the behavioural change: *Commitment*, *Activation*, Taking Steps—abbreviated CAT.

Change talk represents one side of the ambivalence. The other side of the ambivalence is represented by the so-called "sustain talk", which includes all statements in favour of maintaining the status quo.

> Change Talk are all utterances of a client that speak for a change. Sustain Talk are statements that speak for maintaining the status quo.

The aim of the evocation process is to trigger and selectively reinforce change talk. The communication strategies used for this purpose are explained in the following ▶ Sect. 2.8.3. The general aim of an MI conversation is to change the relationship between change talk and sustain talk in the course of the conversation in favour of change talk. The mechanism of action of MI is assumed to be that the counsellor promotes Change Talk through his basic attitude and selective reinforcing communication. As a result, the client hears himself articulate arguments for change. In terms of Bem's (1972) self-perception theory, this perception affects the client's attitudes and beliefs, which in turn influence behavior.

As a final process, the process of planning begins when the client has articulated the motivation for behavior change. The planning process also includes building confidence that the client can bring about the desired change, concretely exploring barriers and resources to goal achievement, and developing a plan to achieve the goal. As mentioned at the beginning, the processes of relationship building, focusing, and evocation are ongoing and will continue to be addressed in the later phases. To illustrate the four processes, Miller and Rollnick's (2013) questions for an MI counselor to ask himself about each process are helpful:

Questions the Counsellor Asks him- or herself with Regard to the 4 Processes of MI (After Miller & Rollnick, 2013, p. 32)

1. Relationship building
   (a) How comfortable is the teenager talking to me?
   (b) How supportive and helpful am I?
   (c) Do I understand the youth's perspective and concerns?
   (d) How comfortable does the conversation feel for me?
   (e) Does it feel like a collaborative partnership?

2. Focus
   (a) What change goals does the adolescent really have?
   (b) Do I have other goals for change for this teen?
   (c) Are we working together with a common cause?
   (d) Does it feel like we're moving together, not in different directions?
   (e) Do I have a clear idea of the direction we are heading?
   (f) Does it feel more like "dancing" or "fighting"?
3. Evocation
   (a) What are the adolescent's reasons for change?
   (b) Is the hesitation more about lack of confidence or lack of importance of change?
   (c) What kind of change talk am I hearing?
   (d) Am I going too far or too fast in a particular direction?
   (e) Does the correction reflex lead me to argue for change?
4. Planning
   (a) What would be a sensible next step towards change?
   (b) What would help this person move in this direction?
   (c) Do I always pay attention to evoking a plan and not prescribing it?
   (d) Do I give needed information and advice with permission?
   (e) Do I maintain an attitude of quiet curiosity about what might work best for this young person?

In all four processes, the counsellor applies certain communication strategies which are at the same time an expression of the MI basic attitude and help to implement the goals of MI. These communication strategies are presented in the following.

2.8.3 OARS

The counsellor supports each of the four described processes of MI with the application of four basic communication strategies with the acronym OARS ("open" questions, "affirmation", "reflection", "summary"), which are meant to support the adolescent in exploring and resolving his ambivalence. The aim here is also to strengthen the young person's decision-making autonomy.

The four basic communication strategies in MI are
1. Ask open questions
2. Affirmation
3. Reflective listening
4. Synopsis

Open-ended questions encourage an open-ended exploration of the adolescent's particular risk behaviour. In contrast to the formulation of closed questions (to which the answer can be yes or no), open questions allow exploration of the reality of the young person's life and encourage contact with the counsellor. They therefore also represent a form of appreciation, in that the counsellor expresses his non-judgemental, authentic interest in the young person's experience and thus conveys that the young person's point of view is taken seriously and is important. In addition, open-ended questions are an important strategy for fostering accurate empathy, as the information thus obtained helps the counselor to take the adolescent's perspective. An open-ended question should always be followed by a series of expressions of reflective listening.

Affirmation includes appreciative recognition and strengthening of the adolescent's resources and all efforts that go in the direction of a change in risk behaviour. For example, in the case of a brief intervention with an alcohol-intoxicated adolescent, this always includes appreciating the adolescent's willingness to talk.

Reflective or active listening is a conversation technique used to learn more about the motives, background and value system of the other person. Often the intention of listening is not to really *understand*, but to respond. In reflective listening, the counselor reflects back to the youth how he or she understood what was said. Active listening promotes the perception of empathy and thereby encourages the young person to feel understood. A distinction can be made between two different forms of reflection: *Simple reflection* reflects what has been said without the counsellor adding meaning or interpretation. *Complex reflection* puts what is said into a different context of meaning or makes assumptions about what might be behind what is said.

Summarising primarily serves to structure the conversation on an ongoing basis and should therefore take place between individual conversation blocks. However, summaries also enable the recurring emphasis of the arguments and motives mentioned by the young person that are significant for a change in behaviour. Here it is important that the young person's perspective is reflected in the summary, i.e. that the reasons for maintaining the status quo (sustain talk) are also considered. However, in terms of MI, the focus should be on summarising the young person's Change Talk. There are summaries with different emphases, e.g., bulleted, linking (relating current Sustain Talk to previously expressed Change Talk), transitioning (transitioning to a new process in MI, e.g., the planning process), or summaries that reflect ambivalence. They should always end with a summary of the Change Talk, since what was said last is often remembered most strongly and clients usually respond to what was said last. In addition, summaries serve to reflect on what was discussed and contribute to clarification. They should always end with an open question.

2.8.4 Dealing with Sustain Talk and Dissonance in the Counsellor-Client Relationship

Miller and Rollnick (2013) abandon their earlier concept of "resistance" in the current edition of MI and replace it with the more nuanced conceptualization of "sustain talk" and dissonance in the counselor-client relationship. Whereas resistance was previously always understood as an expression of a disruption in the counsellor-client relationship, two concepts are now described that can contribute in different ways to the conversation not moving in the direction of change and motivation building.

The first concept mentioned is sustain talk. Sustain Talk is not understood as an expression of intransigence or resistance, but as the natural side of ambivalence. In ambivalence, sometimes the side of wanting change (Change Talk) prevails and sometimes the side of keeping everything as it is (Sustain Talk) . In this, adolescents are no different from adults. With adolescents, there is an additional strong desire to accomplish things on their own. Due to their development, they tend to have a lot of confidence in themselves and distance themselves from offers of help from adults as supposed proof of their lack of independence. In this context, sustain talk is to be understood as the predominance of the side of non-change or as the expression of an intense desire for independence. The side of non-change is partly strengthened by fear or lack of confidence in possible change and possible inner-psychic or interpersonal conflicts. The object and source of Sustain Talk is therefore not the counsellor-client relationship, but the behavioural change itself that is in focus.

In MI, it is assumed that the reasons for sustain talk do not usually need to be explored in depth (exceptions see ▶ Sect. 2.8.5 and point 5 in the box "Strategies for Dealing with Sustain Talk"). Sustain talk is recognised in a value-free way and is seen as a natural part of ambivalence (see ▶ Sect. 2.9). The crucial point is that the counsellor strives to trigger change talk through the targeted use of reflective listening in particular. However, this should not lead to confrontation ("You have fun drinking, but don't you see that…"), but rather the partnership-based, joint perspective of counsellor and client on the risk behaviour should always be maintained.

Strategies for Dealing with Sustain Talk (Miller & Rollnick, 2013)

1. Reflective listening
   (a) simple or complex reflection (often triggers change talk in itself, i.e. argumentation for the other side of the ambivalence)
   (b) exaggerated reflection (slightly exaggerates the intensity of the statement so that change talk is triggered)
   (c) double-sided reflection (acknowledge sustain talk and connect it with previously expressed change talk, connected with "and")
2. Emphasize the autonomy of the young person
3. Refraiming (introducing a new meaning or perspective to what is being said).
4. Agree with turn (reflection + refraiming: first agree, then open a new frame of reference for what is said)
5. "Gaining momentum" (a strategy rarely used and only in cases where almost no Change Talk is articulated: Exploring and acknowledging Sustain Talk in detail first and then getting to the other side of the ambivalence).
6. Agree (without inflection) (also a rather rarely used method in which the counsellor agrees to the sustain talk, possibly with a bit of exaggeration. It is important that this is done without irony).

Dissonance in the therapeutic relationship can be another source of change talk not increasing over the course of the counseling session. Such dissonance can be expressed through arguing, ignoring, interrupting, or downplaying or trivializing and can occur in all four processes of MI (relationship building, focusing, evocation, planning). Sources of dissonance in the therapeutic relationship can be, for example, perceived paternalism by the counsellor or a rash counsellor who already wants to start planning for goal achievement although the client has not yet resolved his ambivalence towards the target behaviour (▶ Sect. 2.9). The same strategies recommended for dealing with sustain talk are used to deal with such situations. In addition, an apology from the counsellor can be helpful in re-establishing an empathic, partnership relationship if, for example, he realises he has been too hasty. Explicit appreciation can also reduce dissonance in the counselor-client relationship. In addition, the counsellor can shift the focus of the conversation and in this way take the tension out of the relationship by steering it towards a new topic.

2.8.5 Dealing with Young People Without Ambivalence

Most people are ambivalent about any harmful behaviour they engage in. Especially with regard to substance use, such as smoking or alcohol consumption, most people are aware of actual and/or potential negative consequences of their behaviour. Working with adolescents is sometimes more challenging in this regard because adolescents typically feel 'invulnerable' and often experience low levels of ambivalence, particularly in relation to alcohol use (Wiers et al., 2007). However, in the case of counselling adolescents following alcohol intoxication, the vast majority of adolescents at least acknowledge treatment in a clinic as a clearly undesirable and negative aspect of drinking. The situation of the counselling interview therefore provides a source for experiencing ambivalence and discrepancy between the status quo and the adolescent's ideas, desires and goals for their own life. It is therefore assumed that the clinic stay represents a so-called "teachable moment" (Lawson & Flocke, 2009), i.e. a moment in which persons are particularly open to health-related information and interventions are particularly effective.

Nevertheless, even in this setting, the counsellor may encounter a young person who does not initially display ambivalence about their alcohol use and who does not express change talk. In these cases, Miller and Rollnick (2013) suggest initially assuming that the young person may experience ambivalence about some aspect of risk behaviour after all. The relationship building process is therefore followed by an in-depth exploration of the young person's internal view of the risk behaviour and an exploration of the young person's values and goals through open-ended questions and reflective listening. The prerequisite for the following phase of focusing is the identification of a discrepancy. Only under this condition can it be decided which behavioural change should be the goal of the conversation. A discrepancy perception, which should lead to an intrinsic motivation to reduce this discrepancy, can only be a discrepancy between current behaviour and personal values and goals of the young person. In this context, the respectful, partnership-based basic attitude in MI enables the young person to recognise and articulate discrepancies without activating mechanisms of self-protection.

In the current conceptualization of MI, Miller and Rollnick (2013) note that, according to recent research, the use of the so-called motivational scale, a four-field scheme that can be used to explore the pros and cons of changing and maintaining behavior (► Fig. 5.6), is contraindicated for individuals with no or very low ambivalence perception, as its use in this case would almost exclusively provoke sustain talk. For individuals whose motivation to change behavior is already high at the time of use, on the other hand, the use of the motivational scale is a suitable tool to further promote Change Talk.

In the case that also in the in-depth exploration no ambivalence and thus no Change Talk was expressed, the counsellor can react with reflective listening. In terms of MI, it is assumed that the counsellor's mirroring of the Sustain Talk can encourage the young person to take the other position (Change Talk). Another strategy of dealing with a young person who does not make statements that move in the direction of change is to share information. Important here is the idea of *exchange*, as opposed to information transfer. Information exchange in MI follows the EPE principle ("elicit"–"provide"–"elicit"), which means ask—give information—ask for. The exchange always starts with an open question to the young person (e.g. "What do you know about alcohol?"). Most young people will already know a fair amount of correct information about underage drinking. This approach avoids the counselor disrupting the empathic and partnership relationship by providing redundant information. Rather, this approach is an expression of genuine interest in the other person and evidence to the adolescent that he or she is being taken seriously. Following this, the counsellor can give information. It is important to ask permission first ("If you agree, I would like to add one more thing…") and to emphasise the young person's autonomy and freedom of choice ("I would like to give you some information on what ideas other young people have had about not putting themselves in danger when they drink. Whether you use this information is, of course, up to you."). The imparting of information is then again followed by reflective listening and open-ended questions to explore the meaning and interpretation of the information given to the young person. ◘ Table 2.3 gives an overview of MI-congruent and -incongruent assumptions with regard to the exchange of information.

◘ **Table 2.3** MI congruent and incongruent assumptions about information exchange (Miller & Rollnick, 2013, p. 138)

MI-incongruent information exchange	**MI congruent information exchange**
I am the expert on why and how a client should change	I have an expertise and the client is an expert on himself
I collect information about problems	I find out what information clients want and need
I correct gaps in knowledge	I adapt information to the needs and strengths of the client
Scary information is helpful	The client can tell me what information is helpful to them
I just need to tell the client clearly what to do	Advice can be helpful if it takes into account the needs and autonomy of the client

Other starting points for triggering change talk may be the request to describe a typical drinking occasion or, if known, the articulation of concern by significant people in the young person's environment. Advice, as a specific form of information, should be given infrequently and only when a good relationship between counselor and client has already been established. At all times, the counselor should ask permission to give advice, while emphasizing the client's autonomy to follow or not follow that advice.

2.9 The Transtheoretical Model of Change According to Prochaska and DiClemente

When working with people who are seeking to change their behaviour, it is helpful to have a theoretical model of human behaviour change. In connection with MI, the transtheoretical model of behavior change according to Prochaska et al. (1992) is typically used to describe the processes that precede behavior change and to be able to adapt therapeutic action accordingly.

The transtheoretical model (TTM) was developed within US clinical psychology in the 1970s. According to the model, the current motivation of a person is considered changeable and influenceable. According to this, a motivation can fluctuate depending on the situation and run in different phases. In contrast to the so-called Rubicon models of behavioural change, the TTM understands behavioural change as a process that passes through various intrapsychic phases of change that precede a visible behavioural change. Rubicon models are two-phase models that assume there is a "threshold" to behavior change. Once the person has crossed this threshold, for example because the distress of not changing has become too great, behaviour change takes place. The TTM, on the other hand, assumes different phases of behavioural change and differentiates them for counselling practice.

According to the TTM, people typically go through five phases to change a particular problem behavior or to start a new behavior and maintain it in a stable manner:

1. Precontemplation,
2. Contemplation,
3. Preparation,
4. Action,
5. Maintenance.

In the *precontemplation phase,* people do not consider changing their behavior in the foreseeable future. They are not receptive to problem-related information, nor do they show attention to cues that might assist in changing behavior. There is no awareness of the problem. This is the most stable of all the stages.

In the *contemplation phase,* there is a possible intention to change. The person becomes open to new insights and observations, to disputes and new interpretations. She begins to rethink her own behavior and anticipate feedback that would be expected from the social environment if she were to change her behavior. The potentially new is also checked against one's own moral evaluations. This self-evaluation allows for the mental preparation and anticipation of an alternative behavior. The person usually remains in this phase for a long time. A change is considered again and again, but postponed. The pros and cons are weighed, creating an underlying ambivalence. In this phase, the costs and benefits of a change in behaviour are difficult for the person to assess.

In the *preparation phase,* the intention to change the harmful behaviour has been made and the first actions towards change are visible. This can manifest itself, for example, in the fact that strategies for a change in behaviour are being considered and already tried out in rudimentary form. This may include activating social support as well as anticipating future situations that make the risky behaviour likely and developing behavioural strategies to avoid the risky behaviour. In this phase of planning, there is a great deal of uncertainty about goal achievement, and strengthening the experience of self-efficacy and activating resources are central to the transition to the next phase.

In the *action phase,* the person has been performing the new behavior regularly for a relatively short time. She usually acts out of an act of self-liberation, this self-awareness being necessary to resist habitual or social temptations. This stage is considered the most difficult. It is advisable to involve support from the social environment, as there is a high probability of relapse.

In the *maintenance phase,* the new behavior is performed and new behavioral habits have formed. Here, too, changes are still possible, but the probability of relapse is lower.

The TTM was developed and tested primarily in connection with addiction problems. It helps the counsellor to adapt his therapeutic behaviour to the respective readiness of the young person to change. For example, working out a target agreement for low-risk alcohol consumption with an adolescent in the absence of intention would trigger reactance and negatively influence the therapeutic relationship. The model also describes that a person can go through the individual phases several times during a change project until a change stabilises (◘ Fig. 2.8).

Relapses are seen as part of the process. The perspective on phases in change processes has also made it possible to take a more differentiated view of the effects of counselling sessions. This is because interventions are to be evaluated as successful even if the client has “only” moved on to the next phase, e.g. from intentionlessness to intention formation.

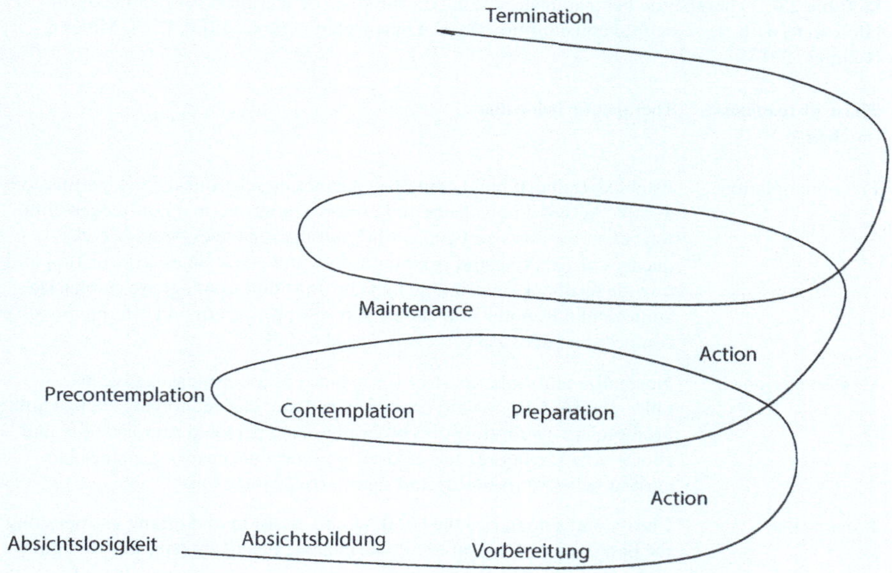

Fig. 2.8 The circular model of the stages of change. (Adapted from Prochaska et al., 1992; this material originally appeared in English as Prochaska, J.O., DiClemente, C.C., & Norcross, J.C. (1992). In search of how people change: Applications to addictive behaviors. American Psychologist, 47(9), 1102–1114. Copyright © 1992 by the American Psychological Association. Translated and reproduced with permission of the publisher and the author. The American Psychological Association is not responsible for the accuracy of this translation. The official citation that should be used in referencing this material is stated above. The use of APA information does not imply endorsement by APA)

2.10 Stages of Readiness for Change and Therapeutic Behaviour

The therapeutic behaviour should always refer to the phase of readiness for change in which the adolescent finds himself. Depending on the adolescent's readiness to change, different emphases are set in the brief motivational intervention in order to trigger optimal motivation to change and to cause as little dissonance as possible in the relationship between counsellor and adolescent. In this way, the counsellor ensures that the young person feels understood and valued and is met where they are at the moment. An overview of appropriate therapeutic behaviour depending on the client's readiness to change is provided in Table 2.4.

Table 2.4 Therapeutic behaviour depending on the stage of readiness for change of an adolescent with risky alcohol consumption (after Dimeff et al., 1999; Miller, 1999; Miller & Rollnick, 2013)

Phase of readiness for change	Therapeutic behaviour
Precontemplation	Establish rapport; build empathic, partnering relationship; ask permission to talk. Accept ambivalence and explore status quo in a non-judgemental way; explore values and goals; work out discrepancies between consequences of drinking and personal values and goals. Share information and provide feedback on drinking habits if the adolescent agrees; emphasize adolescent autonomy and choice. Expressing concern and offering possible contact at a later time if there is a need to talk
Contemplation	Normalize ambivalence; steer the balance of ambivalence (sustain talk—change talk) toward change by evoking and reinforcing change talk; promote intrinsic motivation by emphasizing personal responsibility and choice; focus; reinforce self-efficacy expectations regarding change in current behavior; promote and summarize change talk
Preparation	Clarify and summarize the youth's goals, assist in identifying and selecting the best course of action to initiate change; positively reinforce thoughts and actions toward change, concretize strategies for change, identify possible barriers and helpful resources for dealing with barriers, secure social support
Action	Offer further assistance to the young person, support actions towards change; motivation to and positive reinforcement (appreciation) for the realisation of actions
Maintenance	Communicate relapse prevention strategies

2.11 The Components of the Brief Motivational Intervention According to Spirito et al. (2004)

In 2004, Spirito et al. conducted a study on the effectiveness of brief motivational interventions with adolescents who were treated in an emergency department due to an alcohol-related incident. In this study, the elements of Miller and Rollnick's (2002) motivational interviewing were fleshed out and expanded upon. The motivational interviewing brief intervention conducted by Spirito and coworkers produced reductions in alcohol use among adolescents whose alcohol use had been identified as problematic prior to the clinic visit.

The elements of brief motivational intervention according to Spirito et al. (2004) are:

1. emphasis on personal responsibility;
2. thematisation of drinking motivation and consequences;
3. provision of feedback on consumption patterns and risks;

4. development of different future scenarios in the case of change and non-change;
5. setting goals for future alcohol consumption and
6. establishment of rules for the achievement of objectives.

Important components of the intervention are also the empathic relationship offered by the counsellor and the strengthening of the self-efficacy expectation in the case of Spirito and employees. Points 2–4 also offer starting points for promoting the perception of discrepancies, which is another central aspect of MI.

2.12 Differentiation of Motivational Interviewing from Other Therapeutic Approaches

Motivational interviewing differs from other therapeutic approaches in key elements. According to Miller et al. (1995), this approach differs from cognitive-behavioural therapeutic approaches in, among other things, the assumption that a motivation to change does not necessarily have to be present in relation to the behaviour being discussed, but that triggering an intrinsically motivated intention to change is part of the therapeutic task. Behavioural therapy approaches also teach the client coping strategies and problem-solving skills, while motivational interviewing sees the client as having the competence to develop sustainable change strategies and problem-solving processes.

In contrast to confrontational approaches, motivational interviewing refrains from labeling and the acceptance of certain labels, such as "alcoholic", by the client. Resistance is not understood as a defense with which the client must be confronted, but as an indication of the predominance of one side of the ambivalence (sustain talk) or as an indication of dissonance in the relationship between counselor and client. In both cases, the "non-progress" of the conversation is understood as important feedback for the counsellor, the contents of which can be used for the further course of the conversation.

In contrast to non-directive counselling approaches, the counsellor guides the conversation in MI in a specific direction and specifically reinforces statements made by the client that speak in favour of change (change talk). A clear goal of the motivational interview is formulated by triggering or strengthening the motivation for change. Empathic reflection, as distinguished from non-directive approaches, is used selectively to reinforce change talk. The counsellor may also give advice and information if the client agrees. He therefore does not give neutral advice but is allowed to be transparent about his assessment of the risk behaviour. It is crucial here that the counsellor simultaneously meets the young person's point of view in a non-judgemental way, strives to get to know it as precisely as possible in the spirit of empathy, and always recognises the young person's autonomy in his or her decisions.

The HaLT Hamburg Study

Contents

S. Diestelkamp, R. Thomasius, *Risky Alcohol Consumption among Adolescents*,
https://doi.org/10.1007/978-3-662-68635-5_3

The following chapter describes the development of the brief motivational intervention for children and adolescents with risky alcohol consumption within the framework of the HaLT-Hamburg research project. Besides the study design, the results of the evaluation are presented and discussed.

3.1 Background

HaLT–Hart am LimiT is a nationwide alcohol prevention programme for children and adolescents (Kuttler, 2006; Lang & Kuttler, 2007). The multimodal prevention programme is aimed at minors with risky alcohol consumption and consists of two components. "HaLT proactive" comprises universal prevention measures, the aim of which is to prevent alcohol excesses and harmful alcohol consumption in advance. On the municipal level, the consistent implementation of youth protection is aimed at as well as a broad sensitisation of the public for the promotion of a responsible handling of alcohol. In the module "HaLT reactive", young people who are being treated as inpatients due to acute alcohol intoxication are given the opportunity to take advantage of a brief intervention in the form of a motivating conversation at the bedside ("bridge conversation"). The aim is to reflect on the risky alcohol consumption and to motivate the young person to take part in an experiential group programme ("risk check"). Parents also receive the offer of a counselling session ("parental interview") in the hospital in order to discuss the incident together with a HaLT prevention specialist. The prevention programme HaLT–Hart am LimiT is now carried out at 155 locations nationwide (▶ www.projekt-halt.de). Although the programme is considered 'evidence-informed', no randomised controlled trial (RCT) has yet been available to test the effectiveness of the brief motivational bedside intervention compared with standard hospital treatment. This was done in the HaLT Hamburg study.

3.2 Development of the HaLT Hamburg Intervention

The brief motivational intervention in the HaLT-Hamburg project was developed based on the guideline and conversation guide for the bridge conversation of the HaLT—Hart am LimiT programme (Villa Schöpflin, 2009, 2010) and with the inclusion of international research findings at the German Center for Addiction Research in Childhood and Adolescence (DZSKJ). In the course of developing the intervention manual, a systematic literature search was conducted in ten international databases [Medline, EMBASE, PubMed, Science Citation Index Expanded & Social Sciences Citation Index (Web of Science), PsycInfo, Database of Abstracts of Reviews and Effects (DARE), CINAHL, Cochrane Clinical Trials & Cochrane Database of Systematic Reviews, Psyndex, and Current Controlled Trials] on research findings on brief interventions for at-risk alcohol-using children and adolescents in emergency settings were conducted (Diestelkamp et al., 2016). The literature thus compiled was analysed in a second step with regard to intervention elements for which a relationship with intervention effectiveness was theoretically assumed and/or empirically found. Existing manuals such as the *BASICS—Brief Alcohol Screening and Intervention of College Students* (Dimeff et al., 1999), *Motivational Enhancement*

Therapy Manual (Miller et al., 1995), and the *Treatment Improvement Protocol (TIP) Series 35* (Miller, 1999) and their evaluation results were analyzed in terms of elements of the intervention that were derived from theory and/or whose integration was shown to increase effectiveness. In a next step, a raw version of the HaLT Hamburg intervention manual was created from this theory- and empirically-guided pool of relevant elements, which in the following weeks was transferred into a working version in a participatory consensual process involving the practice partners (addiction counselling for children, adolescents and relatives Kö16a, drug and alcohol outpatient clinic for adolescents, young adults and their families (DAA) at the University Medical Center Hamburg-Eppendorf). Here, attention was paid to the integration of elements of the guideline and conversation guide for the bridge conversation of the programme HaLT–Hart am LimiT (Villa Schöpflin, 2009) in order to ensure the generalizability of the results of the HaLT Hamburg study to the HaLT–Hart am LimiT bridge conversation.

3.3 Study Design

In a randomized-controlled study with two groups (intervention and control group) the effectiveness of the HaLT-Hamburg intervention was investigated. Data collection in the hospitals (t_0) took place from mid-July 2011 to mid-January 2014 on the Friday, Saturday and Sunday morning after alcohol intoxication in each of the six participating Hamburg hospitals (Altonaer Kinderkrankenhaus, Asklepios Klinik Altona, Asklepios Klinik Nord—Heidberg, Helios Mariahilf Klinik, Katholisches Kinderkrankenhaus Wilhelmstift and Universitätsklinikum Hamburg-Eppendorf). Three and six months after the first data collection, a follow-up telephone survey was conducted (t_1, t_2). Prior to this, a framework agreement was concluded with the representatives of the statutory health insurance funds in a cooperation between the Hamburg Authority for Health and Consumer Protection (BGV) and the statutory health insurance funds to remunerate the HaLT Hamburg counsellors on a fee basis.

Patients were eligible to participate in the study if the following criteria were met:

A. inpatient admission for alcohol intoxication,
B. age under 18,
C. sufficient knowledge of German to understand the contents of the examination,
D. no serious physical injury that could massively affect the implementation.

For organisational reasons, randomisation was carried out for one hospital per weekend ("cluster randomisation"). If the control condition was implemented in the hospital on the corresponding day, data collection was carried out on site by a member of the evaluation team alone. In addition, adolescents in the control condition received standard medical care and were given a folder with information on risky alcohol consumption in adolescence and contact details of the cooperating youth-specific addiction counselling centre (Kö16a) ("treatment as usual", TAU). If, on the other hand, the implementation of the intervention condition was successful in the hospital on that day, a counsellor of the mobile intervention team was additionally contacted by the member of the evaluation team, who then carried out the intervention at the bedside and the parental interview (◘ Fig. 3.1). Adolescents in the intervention group also received a telephone booster 6 weeks after the intervention

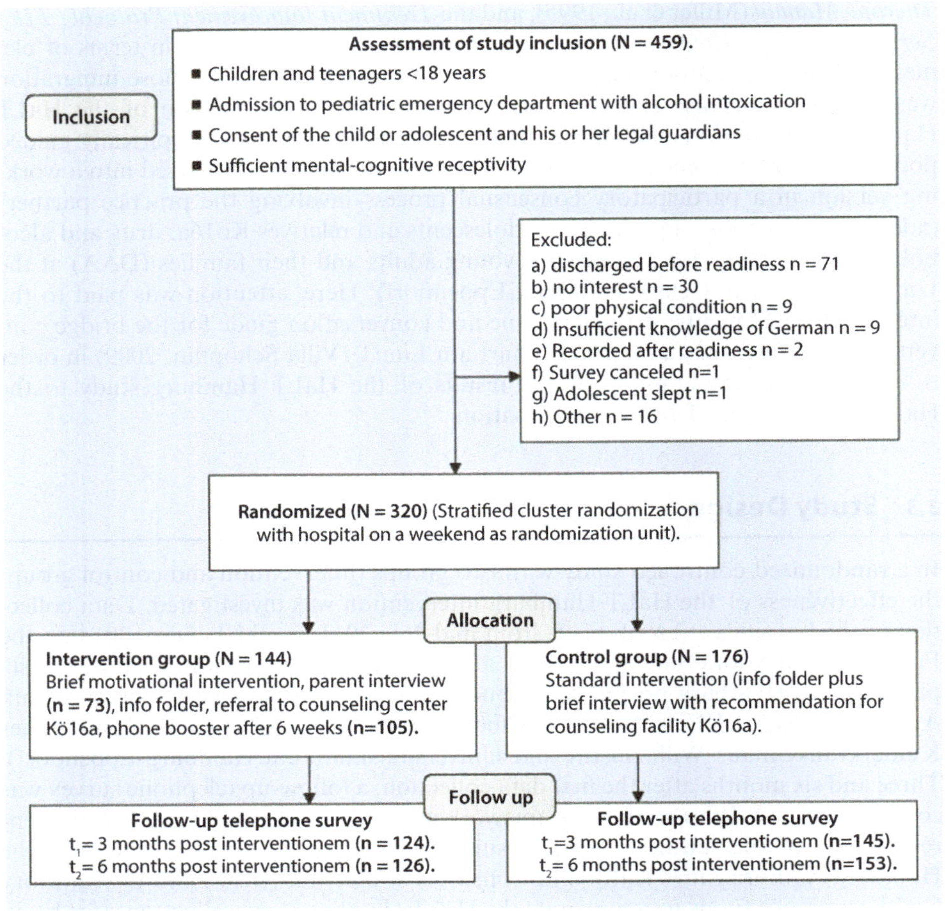

Fig. 3.1 CONSORT study flow chart

(▶ Fig. 5.11). A detailed description of the study design can be found in Diestelkamp et al. (2014).

The study tested the hypotheses that adolescents in the intervention group would reduce their alcohol consumption (number of binge drinking episodes in the past 30 days, number of standard drinks at a typical drinking occasion) and their alcohol-related problems more after the intervention than adolescents in the control group (primary hypotheses). In addition, it was hypothesized that adolescents in the intervention group would more often accept further counseling services than adolescents in the control group (secondary hypothesis).

3.3.1 Measuring Instruments

Data were collected at all three measurement points using standardised questionnaires. The substance history (consumption of alcohol and illicit substances) was taken according to the standards of the German Society for Addiction Research and Addiction Therapy. Alcohol-related problems were assessed by means of an abbreviated version of the Rutgers Alcohol Problems Index (RAPI; Earleywine et al., 2008). Using the screening instruments CRAFFT-d (Tossmann et al., 2009) and RAFFT (Laging, 2005) were used to assess risky alcohol and drug use. In addition, the readiness to change was assessed using the Stages of Change Algorithm (Heidenreich & Hoyer, 2001) and the Screening of Mental Disorders in Adolescence (SPS-J) (Hampel & Petermann, 2005). A detailed description of the instruments used can be found in Diestelkamp et al. (2014).

3.3.2 Statistical Analyses

All statistical analyses described below were performed using SPSS software, version 20 (IBM SPSS, 2011). Cross-sectional comparisons of adolescents in the intervention and control groups were made to describe the sample, using t-tests for independent samples for continuous variables and chi-square tests for categorical variables. Longitudinal analyses were conducted using linear mixed models to test the three primary questions and a mixed logistic model for the secondary question. The significance level chosen was 0.05 in accordance with standard conventions.

3.4 Evaluation Results

3.4.1 Who Does HaLT-Hamburg Reach? Description of the Sample

A total of 316 children and adolescents under the age of 18 (and 169 parents), each treated for acute alcohol intoxication at one of the six Hamburg clinics with pediatric emergency care on a weekend between 2011 and 2014, participated in the HaLT-Hamburg study. Participants were on average 15.8 years old at baseline, with 141 assigned to the intervention group and 175 to the control group. Valid data were available from 281 participants (89%) at the third interview time point after 6 months.

129 young people could not be interviewed, although the young people would presumably have met the inclusion criteria. The non-participation of these young people in the survey was most often due to organisational reasons (e.g. dismissal of the person before the arrival of the project staff); a small percentage (30 cases in total) refused to take part in the survey because there was no interest in participating (◘ Fig. 3.2).

The intervention group and the control group differed statistically significantly in only a few parameters. In the intervention group, a higher percentage of the adolescents had a father with a migration background. Furthermore, more adolescents in the intervention group reported problem drug use compared to the control group. In all other parameters of sociodemography and substance use as well as psychological distress, there were no differences between the two groups, which can be interpreted as evidence of successful random assignment.

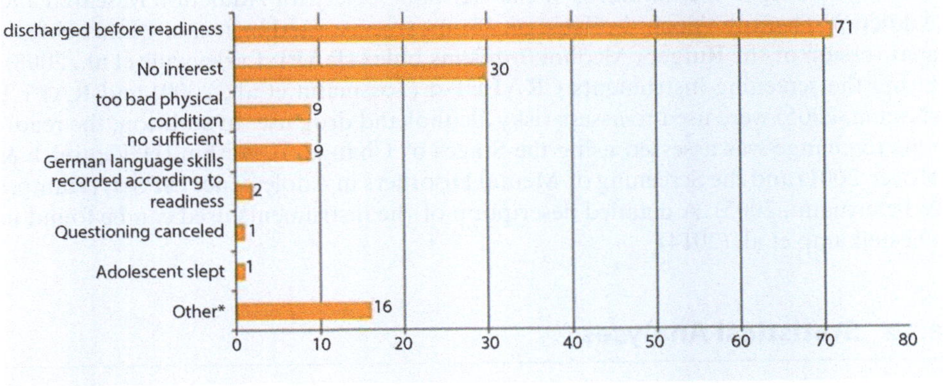

Fig. 3.2 Reasons for non-participation in the HaLT Hamburg study (frequencies)

For the total group, the high percentage of children and adolescents with problematic alcohol consumption was particularly remarkable, as well as the substantial proportion with problematic drug use. 63% were above the cut-off value of the CRAFFT-d screening for risky alcohol consumption in adolescence and 25% above the cut-off value for problematic drug use in the RAFFT screening. (Table 3.1).

Latent class analysis was also used to identify subgroups with different drinking patterns and associated psychosocial problems:

1. low risk consumption (61.2%);
2. risky consumption (21.5%);
3. high-risk consumption (16.5%).

These risk groups could be validly assigned by the screening instruments used (CRAFFT-d and RAPI). The results also show the heterogeneity of the population of alcohol-intoxicated children and adolescents and have implications for an individualised design of measures of indicated prevention as well as for an optimised referral to further treatment or counselling (Diestelkamp et al., 2015).

3.4.2 Effectiveness of Brief Motivational Intervention at the Bedside

Study participants in both the intervention (IG) and control (KG) groups significantly reduced their alcohol consumption and alcohol-related problems following clinic attendance. The reductions were substantial and more pronounced in the IG than in the KG; however, the differences between the two groups were not statistically significant. At the 3-month follow-up, the number of binge drinking episodes in the last 30 days decreased by 62.1% in the intervention group (−1.36, 95% confidence interval CI −1.81 to −0.91) and by 49.0% in the control group (−1.29, 95% CI −1.77 to −0.95). Similar values were reported for the 6-month follow-up (Fig. 3.3). However, these differences between groups were not statistically significant (*p*-values: 0.780 and 0.731).

Table 3.1 Characteristics of the study participants

Parameter	
Age (years)	15.76
Gender	♂: 52%; ♀: 48%
School attendance	Yes: 90%; No: 10%
Mother not born in Germany	Yes: 24%; No: 77%
Father not born in Germany	Yes: 28%; No: 72%
Age at first consumption of alcohol (years)	13.22
Regular alcohol consumption in the last 12 months (at least one time per week)	Yes: 22%; No: 78%
Age at first use of tobacco (years)	13.02
Regular tobacco use in the last 12 months (daily use)	Yes: 35%; No: 65%
Age at first use of cannabis (years)	14.07
Regular cannabis use in the last 12 months (at least ten times per year)	Yes: 20%; No: 80%
Problematic alcohol consumption	Yes: 63%; No: 37%
Problematic drug use	Yes: 25%; No: 75%
Previously in the hospital due to alcohol intoxication.	Yes: 10%; No: 90%
Average number of binge drinking episodes in the last 30 days	2.37
Average number of standard drinks consumed on a typical consumption day	6.49

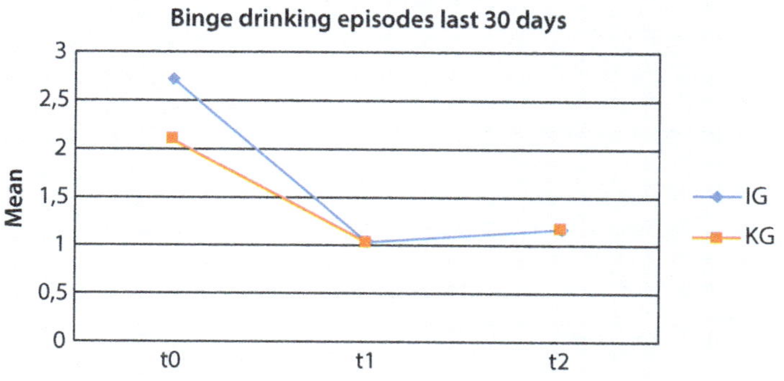

Fig. 3.3 Mean values of the number of binge drinking episodes in the last 30 days across the measurement time points in the intervention (IG) and control (KG) groups

The number of standard drinks per day of consumption also decreased significantly over time for both groups (p-values ranging from 0.011 to <0.001) (◘ Fig. 3.4). In the intervention group, the number reduced by an average of 37.5% (−2.24, 95% CI, −3.18 to −1.29), and in the control group by 26.4% (−1.34, 95% CI −2.54 to −0.14). However, no statistically significant differences were observed between the intervention and control groups (p-values: 0.274 and 0.808).

A similar picture emerged for the third primary outcome. Comparing the first measurement point with the second or third measurement point, both groups (intervention and control group) showed statistically significant time effects for the reduction of alcohol-related problems ($p < 0.001$) (◘ Fig. 3.5). Again, there were no

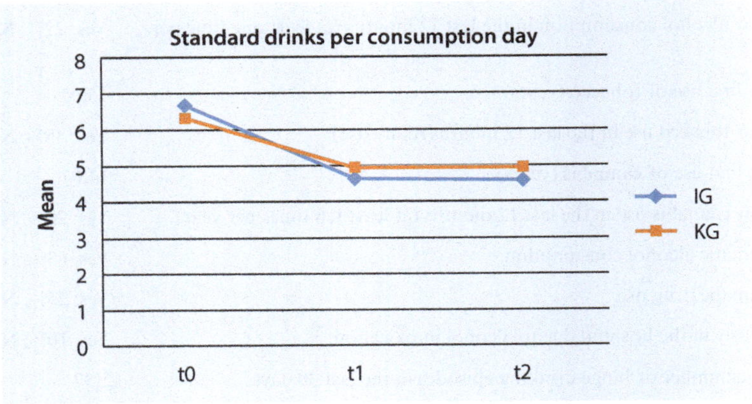

◘ **Fig. 3.4** Mean values of the number of standard drinks consumed at a typical drinking occasion across the measurement time points in the intervention (IG) and control (KG) groups

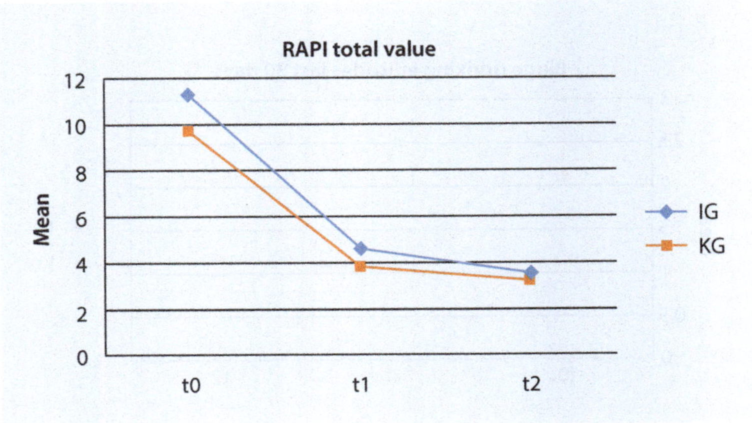

◘ **Fig. 3.5** Mean scores for alcohol-related problems in the last 3 months across measurement time points in the intervention (IG) and control (KG) groups

statistically significant differences between the intervention and control groups (p-values: 0.606 and 0.904). At 3-month follow-up, adolescents in the IG reported 60.5% fewer alcohol-related problems (−6.72, 95% CI −7.68 to −5.76), whereas adolescents in the control group reported 58.3% fewer alcohol-related problems (−6.43, 95% CI, −7.37 to −5.49).

Participants in the IG also made more frequent use of further counselling and treatment services (27% vs. 23% at t_1). Here too, however, the difference to the KG was not significant. In addition to the central analyses, post-hoc analyses were also conducted for the primary questions. For this purpose, we examined whether the variables age, gender, positive screening result for problematic alcohol consumption at t_0 (CRAFFT-d) and psychosocial stress (SPS-J) had a statistically significant influence on the reported results in extended mixed linear models. There was no significant moderating influence of these variables on the results of the three primary questions and the secondary question.

3.4.3 Positive Appreciation by the Counsellor Promotes Readiness to Change

In order to gain further insights into the mechanisms of action of the brief intervention, counsellor and intervention variables were analysed. To this end, the influence of various counsellor variables (empathy, appreciation, competence, congruence) and intervention variables (use of the importance and confidence scale, motivational scales, written target agreement) on the motivation to change in order to reduce alcohol consumption was examined. In a multiple regression analysis, higher levels of the basic therapeutic skill "positive regard" ($R^2 = 7.1\%$; $p < 0.01$) and ending the intervention with a written goal agreement ($R^2 = 2.9\%$; $p < 0.05$) were found to be significant predictors of higher motivation to change. Lower adolescent age ($R^2 = 10.2\%$; $p < 0.01$) was also associated with higher readiness to change (Diestelkamp et al., 2016).

3.4.4 Process Evaluation: The HaLT-Hamburg Project from the Counsellors' Point of View

In addition to the core analyses of effectiveness, qualitative and quantitative surveys were conducted on the accessibility, feasibility, practicality, and acceptability of the intervention in the clinic context (Arnaud et al., 2015). This involved interviewing counsellors involved in implementation ($N = 5$), clinic staff in the emergency context ($N = 39$) and ward managers ($N = 6$), as well as young people who had received an intervention ($N = 144$).

In summary, the survey showed that the intervention was feasible with a high level of acceptance (e.g. acceptable effort, few interface problems between counsellors and clinic staff, etc.) on the part of the actors involved and a high level of satisfaction on

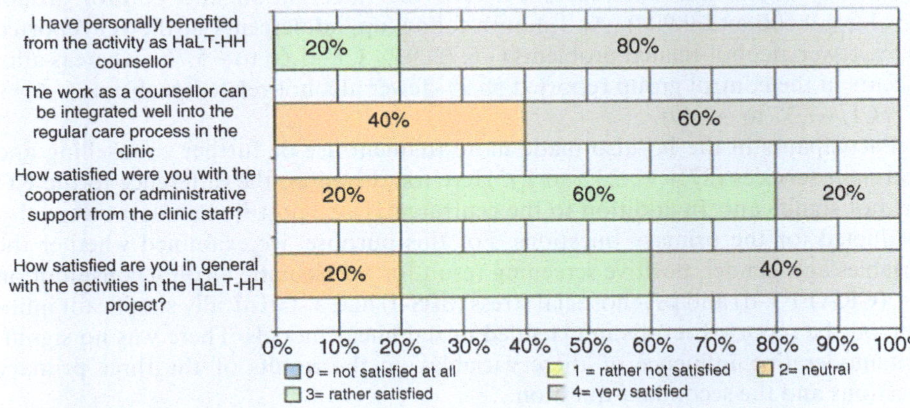

Fig. 3.6 Satisfaction with and feasibility of the HaLT-Hamburg project from the perspective of HaLT-Hamburg counsellors

the part of the patients in the setting, could be integrated well into the regular processes in the clinics and improved the care of alcohol-intoxicated children and adolescents and their parents from the point of view of those involved (Fig. 3.6).

3.4.5 The HaLT-Hamburg Project from the Perspective of Hospital Staff and Chief Physicians

The involvement of hospital staff in the implementation of HaLT-Hamburg primarily concerned telephone coordination with HaLT-Hamburg counsellors (first naming of a total of 23 staff members), providing premises and informing the counsellors about the patients' condition.

Overall, both the head physicians and the clinic staff directly involved in the HaLT-Hamburg intervention were generally satisfied or very satisfied with the project and the cooperation with the counsellors and rated the feasibility in the emergency setting as high or very high. The chief physicians consistently stated that their clinic would benefit from HaLT-Hamburg, that the implementation of the intervention could be carried out with little effort on their part, and that it could be integrated well into regular procedures without interfering with them (Fig. 3.7).

This positive assessment was largely shared by the hospital staff directly involved in the implementation of HaLT-Hamburg, even if the approval rates here were not quite as high as among the head physicians. There was agreement that HaLT-Hamburg improved the care of alcohol-intoxicated adolescents and their parents and that the activities of the HaLT-Hamburg counsellors could be well integrated into the processes on the ward (Fig. 3.8).

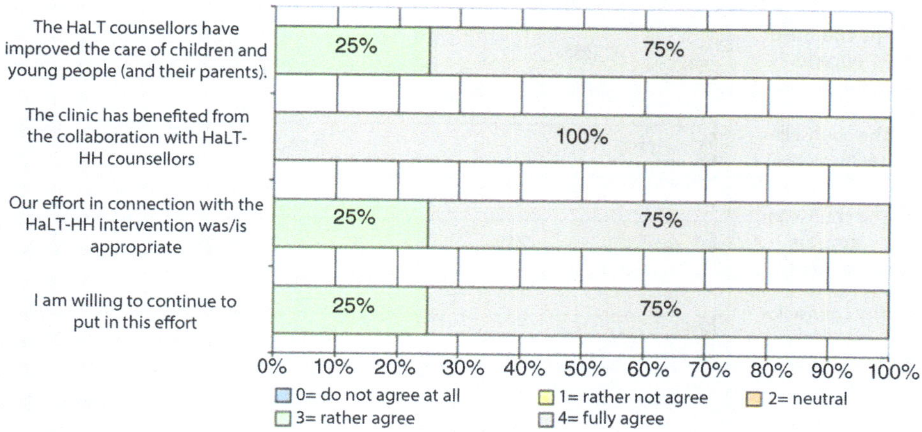

Fig. 3.7 Assessment of the suitability of HaLT-Hamburg for practice by chief physicians

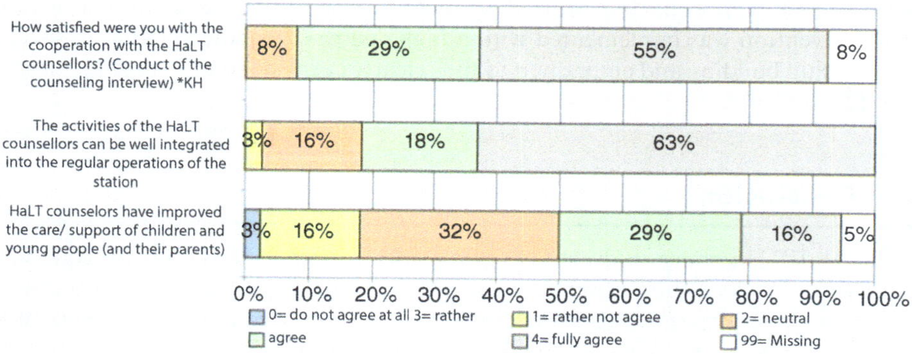

Fig. 3.8 Assessment of satisfaction with and practical suitability of HaLT-Hamburg by the participating clinic staff

3.4.6 Assessment of Therapeutic Relationship Behaviour from the Perspective of the Study Participants

All 141 children and adolescents who had received the brief motivational intervention as part of the study were surveyed following the intervention regarding their perceptions of the counsellor. For this purpose, the "basic therapeutic skills" scale of the needs-oriented interaction scales (BIS) (Stucki, 2002) was used to elicit the 4 dimensions "empathy", "congruence", "positive regard" and "expertise" of thera-

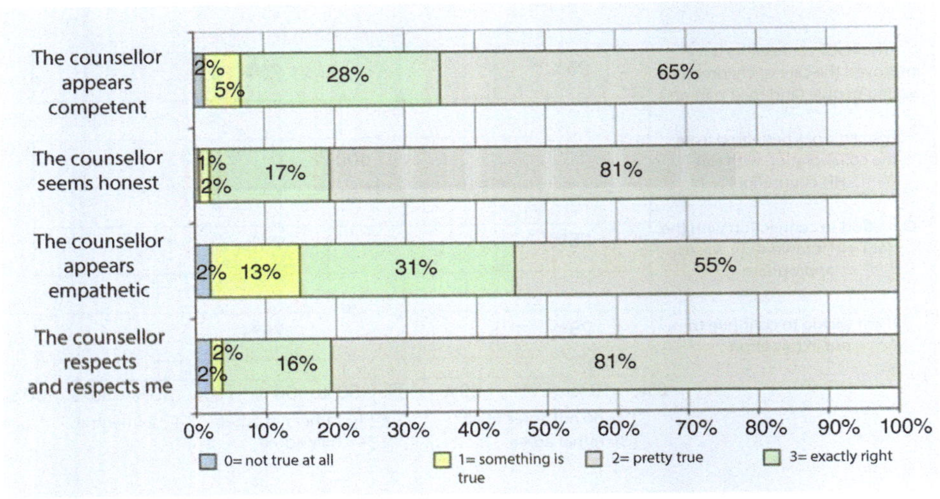

Fig. 3.9 Assessment of therapeutic relationship behaviour from the patient's perspective

peutic relationship behaviour from the patient's perspective. The results suggest that the intervention was implemented with a high degree of partnership and respectful relationship building and empathy, and thus clearly corresponded to the basic idea of MI (Fig. 3.9).

3.5 Conclusion

In the HaLT-Hamburg study, study participants in both groups reported significant reductions in alcohol consumption and alcohol-related problems 3 and 6 months after clinic attendance, which were mostly most pronounced in the contrast between the in-clinic interview (t_0) and after 3 months (t_1), but persisted after 6 months. The number of binge drinking episodes per month decreased by an average of 1.4 episodes (IG to t_1) and the number of standard drinks per day of consumption decreased by 1.8 standard drinks (IG to t_1). Self-reported alcohol-related problems also decreased substantially. Consistently lower levels of these variables were observed in the intervention group than in the control group. It was also found that participants in the intervention group had sought further counselling more frequently than participants in the KG. However, the reductions in the intervention group did not differ significantly from the reductions in the control group.

The approach of treating alcohol-intoxicated children and adolescents with psychosocial interventions while they are still in hospital is often justified by the fact that the situational context (alcohol-related hospitalization) is accompanied by an increased sensitivity for a therapeutic approach, a so-called "teachable moment" (TM). This widely used conceptualization of TM (Spirito et al., 2004; Kuttler, 2006) contrasts with an alternative conceptualization that assumes that the occurrence of a health-related event (e.g., hospitalization) can in itself lead to behavior change

(Lawson & Flocke, 2009; McBride et al., 2003). A possible explanation for the fact that both groups in the HaLT Hamburg study reduced their consumption after hospitalization could be that intoxication in connection with hospitalization represented such a health-relevant event, which led to spontaneous behavioral changes in both groups.

Another possible explanation for the findings could be that the interview and personal contact with a member of the evaluation team triggered possible reflection processes and thus a reduction in consumption in the control group (interview and attention effects). Such effects have been widely documented in the literature (Heather, 2014; McCambridge & Kypri, 2011; Bischof et al., 2012) and would imply that the true effects of the intervention were underestimated under study conditions. For ethical reasons, it was not possible in the HaLT Hamburg study to set up a so-called "no-contact" control group, which does not receive any questioning or information during the clinic stay.

While the effectiveness of brief alcohol interventions is generally well established, the evidence for their effectiveness in adolescence is still mixed (► Sect. 2.7). One possible explanation for this could be that automatic, impulsive processes in behaviour control are clearly more influential in adolescence than in later adulthood. In line with the dual process model of adolescent risk behaviour according to Wiers et al. (2010); ► Sect. 2.4.3), it is assumed that a motivational intervention strengthens both motivation and the capacity for self-control and thus has a moderating effect on impulsive processes. Given the particularly influential nature of impulsive processes on risk behaviours, especially in early and middle adolescence (Steinberg, 2010), it is conceivable that a one-off bedside intervention with a brief telephone booster after 6 weeks may not be intensive enough to sustainably strengthen motivation and ability to self-control. For this age group, complementary developmentally specific services might need to be developed to provide closer follow-up, for example through a smartphone app. Overall, the HaLT Hamburg study was able to show that a relevant target group can be reached with an offer that meets with a high level of acceptance through the counselling session in the hospital.

Practice

Contents

S. Diestelkamp, R. Thomasius, *Risky Alcohol Consumption among Adolescents*, https://doi.org/10.1007/978-3-662-68635-5_4

Based on the theoretical foundation described in ▶ Chap. 2, the practical part of this manual provides detailed instructions for the procedure and implementation of the brief motivational intervention at the bedside and for the parent interview.

After explaining the theoretical background on which the brief motivational intervention is based and the evaluation results of the HaLT-Hamburg study, the practical implementation of the intervention at the bedside is now described below. The intervention is described as it was implemented and evaluated in the HaLT-Hamburg research project. New recommendations that can be derived from the updated conceptualization of MI by Miller and Rollnick (2013) are referred to in corresponding footnotes.

First, the goals to be achieved with the intervention are explained. Then the course of the intervention is presented in detail and necessary preparations for the implementation of the session are named. Then the implementation of the intervention is described with its parts "welcome and presentation of the project", "brief motivational intervention adolescents", "parent interview", "final interview" and "documentation".

4.1 Practical Implementation of the HaLT Hamburg Intervention

4.1.1 Target Group

The target group for the HaLT-Hamburg intervention are children and adolescents who are hospitalized due to acute alcohol intoxication. The intervention is specifically aimed at minors and therefore addresses all adolescents up to the age of 18. At the time of the interview with the counsellor, the young person must have sufficient mental-cognitive receptivity and sufficient German language comprehension to be able to participate in the intervention.

4.1.2 Qualifications of the Counsellors

In the HaLT-Hamburg research project, social pedagogues, psychologists, pedagogues, educationalists and physicians could act as counsellors, preferably having started or completed additional therapeutic training and/or addiction-specific training. Before taking up their work, the HaLT-Hamburg counsellors received a 1.5-day training in the implementation of the manualised brief motivational intervention. During their work as HaLT-Hamburg counsellors, participation in regular supervisions every 2 months was obligatory.

4.1.3 General Conditions

If possible, the participating clinics provide a room for the implementation of the intervention in which the discussions can take place in an undisturbed atmosphere. All materials required for the implementation of the intervention are attached to this manual.

Table 4.1 Schedule of the brief motivational intervention at the bedside with time details

Time	Content
10 min	Welcome and presentation of the project
45 min	Brief motivational intervention adolescents
30 min	Parent intervention
10 min	Final interview
10 min	Documentation

4.1.4 Procedure

Depending on local agreements, the cooperating clinic informs the counsellor on duty about the admission of an underage patient diagnosed with acute alcohol intoxication. In the HaLT-Hamburg study, active contacting of the counsellors to the clinics has proven successful. Depending on the available personnel resources at the locations, it is recommended to define on-call times. The highest treatment numbers were observed in a Hamburg pilot study at weekends (Saturday and Sunday mornings), and to a lesser extent on Friday mornings (Sack et al., 2009). The evaluation of case numbers at 24 Hamburg clinics over a period of 1 year did not reveal any accumulations of treatment numbers on public holidays, special major events or, for example, at the beginning of holidays. In the HaLT Hamburg study, a mobile intervention team was on call Friday to Sunday between 7 and 9 a.m.[1]

After arriving at the hospital, the counsellor visits the young person in his or her room. He or she introduces him-/ herself and the matter at hand (cf. "Greeting and introduction of the matter at hand"). If the parents or guardians have already arrived, the counsellor also introduces him/herself to them and explains the content, procedure and aims of the counselling offer and obtains the adolescent's consent to participate in the brief intervention and that of the parents in the parental interview. Table 4.1 gives an overview of the course of the intervention with details of the intended duration of the individual parts.

The counsellor then conducts the brief motivational intervention with the young person, which lasts about 45 min and aims to reflect on the circumstances of the alcohol intoxication and to trigger and strengthen intrinsic motivation to reduce the risk of future alcohol consumption (► Sect. 4.4.2). Where possible, the interview should be conducted in a room with adequate privacy and not in the presence of parents. Assurance of the confidentiality of the contents of the conversation is central to establishing an open atmosphere for the conversation and thus a prerequisite for implementing the spirit of MI.

A discussion is then held with the parents or guardians of the young person. At the end of the respective conversation, the parents and the adolescent receive the recommendation to take advantage of a further counselling offer in an addiction

1 Information on young people reached and not reached during these periods 7 Sect. 3.4.1.

counselling centre. In addition, the young person is given the HaLT Hamburg information folder, which contains information on rules for low-risk alcohol consumption and an information brochure from a local addiction counselling centre.

Six weeks after the bedside intervention in the HaLT Hamburg study, a telephone contact was made with all adolescents who had consented to this. The aim of this so-called telephone booster was to refresh the motivation established in the hospital for low-risk consumption and to address possible obstacles to achieving the goals formulated in the clinic. If goals were achieved, motivation to maintain the desired behavior was strengthened and strategies for relapse prevention were discussed. If the goals were not achieved, possible barriers and resources for achieving the goals were discussed again and the counselling services of the local addiction counselling centre were pointed out (▶ Fig. 5.11).

4.1.5 Preparations

On days when the counsellor is on call for the mobile intervention team, he or she will have the following ready for his assignments:

- Cell Phone,
- Telephone list of the intervention team counsellors on duty,
- Fact Sheet Deployment Information,
- Memo Cards,
- Consumables in sufficient quantity:
  - HaLT Hamburg interview,
  - Motivational Scale Template,
  - Importance and confidence scale template,
  - Template target agreement youth,
  - Template Target Agreement Parents,
  - Pens,
  - Interview documentation for counsellors,
  - HaLT-Hamburg information folder for young people.

Depending on how familiar the counsellor already is with the materials, he or she will visualise the course of the intervention once again before the start of the intervention and, in particular, go through the HaLT Hamburg interview and the memo cards in order to facilitate a smooth process on site.

4.2 Objectives of the Brief Motivational Intervention for Adolescents

The primary goal of the brief intervention is to reach adolescents who have already attracted attention due to their admission to a clinic at an early stage, in order to support them in developing a responsible and conscious approach to alcohol, without being stigmatising or moralising and thereby provoking resistance ("reactance") to the use of counselling services. Rather, the brief intervention aims to establish an initial relationship with the young person. Among other things, the young person should be made aware of the fact that the behaviour shown is a cause for concern and the problematic behaviour should be pointed out in an empathetic way, which may not be perceived as such by the young person himself, for instance if the majority of the immediate peer group shows a similar pattern of use. It is also important to adopt a differentiated attitude towards the young person and to signal that it is not a question of addiction or the awarding of a diagnosis, but of risky consumption behaviour. The aim is to trigger and promote the young person's perception of ambivalence with regard to his or her alcohol consumption and to trigger and promote motivation for low-risk consumption.

An overview of the aims of the brief motivational intervention with the adolescent are:

- Encourage reflection on alcohol intoxication and accompanying circumstances,
- Stimulating a differentiated examination of one's own alcohol consumption patterns,
- Elaboration and clarification of ambivalences in relation to dealing with alcohol,
- Promote intrinsic motivation to change behavior,
- Establish goals related to low-risk use of alcohol and strategies for achieving them,
- Motivation to seek further counselling.

The brief motivational intervention is divided into the phases of conversation initiation, semi-structured interview, exploration, summarizing and clarifying, and conversation conclusion. The memo card "Brief Motivational Intervention Adolescents" is used at the bedside, which is used by the HaLT-Hamburg counsellors during the intervention as an orientation aid for the structure and content of the intervention (▶ Fig. 5.2).

4.3 Goals of the Parent Intervention

The intervention with the parents or guardians of the adolescents aims to develop a basis for the future support of the adolescent in pursuing his or her goal of risk reduction in dealing with alcohol. This is based on the concept for parent training of young people at risk of addiction according to Stolle et al. (2010), which is divided into the components

1. Recognition,
2. Understanding and
3. Support.

Parents are given information about alcohol consumption among adolescents, which enables them to better assess whether their son's or daughter's alcohol consumption is typical adolescent experimental consumption or harmful use, or whether there is a possible risk of addiction. In addition, possible motivations for the adolescent's risky alcohol use are discussed and strategies for supporting the adolescent are developed. If the adolescent does not intend to change his or her use of alcohol, the parents are taught the principles of motivational interviewing, if they are interested, which should enable them to remain in conversation with the adolescent without provoking the adolescent to break off communication by triggering reactance.

4.4 Implementation of the Brief Motivational Intervention

4.4.1 Welcome and Presentation of the Project

The first contact with the young person and the guardians primarily serves to introduce the counsellor, the project and to clarify the willingness to participate. This introductory part of the intervention is at the same time indicative for the further course of the intervention, since the relationship building already begins with the first contact.

Objectives "Welcome and Presentation of the Project"

- Provide an overview of the process and objectives of the intervention
- Trigger willingness to participate in the project
- Gathering initial information
- Beginning of the establishment of rapport or relationship building

In preparation for the intervention, the counsellor should therefore be aware of the basic therapeutic attitude he or she wishes to adopt towards his interlocutors before each initial meeting with a young person and the guardians. Already in the greeting, his attitude of appreciation, respect and empathic, partnership relationship offer should become clear. The counsellor conveys his or her attitude indirectly through non-judgmental reflective listening and directly through the expression of appreciation regarding individual behaviours. An authentic start to the conversation and the establishment of empathy, above all through positive reinforcement and recognition of the young person's willingness to talk, form the basis for willingness to participate and for the conversation that follows. The counsellor shows interest in the young person and expresses concern about the current behaviour.

Counsellor:	"Good day, my name is (...) and I am a staff member of the HaLT-Hamburg project. We come to the Hamburg clinics when a young person with alcohol intoxication has been admitted to the clinic to have a talk with him and his parents. May I give you some information about this?"
Parents:	"Yes, of course"
Counsellor:	(to the youth) "Is it all right with you?"
Adolescent:	"Yeah, why not"

At this point, the counsellor clarifies whether the young person would like to be addressed as "Sie" or "Du". Young people over the age of 16 should generally be addressed as "Du", but the counsellor should always ask and choose the form of address that the young person prefers.

Counsellor: "First of all, I want to express my appreciation to you for taking the time to pick up your son and for being willing (to the teenager) to listen to why I am here. The fact that you were admitted to the hospital yesterday certainly worries all of you a lot and you worry a lot. In recent years, more and more young people are finding that they cannot control their alcohol consumption and have to be treated in hospital with alcohol poisoning. That's why the HaLT-Hamburg project exists, offering support to young people if they want to avoid such incidents in the future"

In this introductory part of the interview, the counsellor shows interest, concern and empathy for what has happened and for those involved. Right at the beginning he asks for permission to give the guardians and the adolescent information about the project and thus triggers an initial commitment to participate in the conversation, thus reducing the risk that resistance[2] will arise at this stage. It is important that the counsellor includes the young person as an equal partner in the conversation from the outset and addresses him or her, thus avoiding the impression that this is a conversation between adults about the young person. The counsellor expresses appreciation for the willingness to hear information about the project and for the parents' commitment to their child. He or she may also comment appreciatively on other aspects at this point if he has noticed indications of this in the brief contact so far. The more individual the reference to the interlocutor, the more empathetic the interlocutor feels accepted and the more authentic the resulting relationship. The counsellor responds to resistance[3] by reflecting, shifting the focus, agreeing with a twist, emphasising personal freedom of choice, reinterpreting or conforming (▶ Sect. 2.8.4).

Parents: (upset) "We don't need any information. We've already talked him into it and it won't happen again because he's banned from going out from now on anyway"

Counsellor: "I can see that you are very concerned about your son and that you care very much that such an incident does not happen again. That is our concern as well and I would like to talk with you and with your son about how exactly you would like to accomplish this. How does that sound to you?"

From the answer to the question whether the adolescent is interested in information about the offered conversation, you already get a first impression of the readiness for change that the adolescent has regarding his handling of alcohol. Depending on the readiness for change that the young person signals, the counsellor chooses a different conversation starter to motivate the young person to take part in the conversation.

---

2 According to Miller and Rollnick (2013), this would be referred to as dissonance in the counselor-client relationship.

3 According to Miller and Rollnick (2013), this would be referred to as sustain talk and dissonance in the counselor-client relationship.

▶ Example 1

Adolescent: (expresses no need for change to the counsellor and signals no willingness to cooperate).

Counsellor: "I can understand that after such a night, you don't feel like having a conversation about today's incident. May I still explain to you what the conversation should be about?"

▶ Example 2

Adolescent: (Expresses shock to the counsellor about the incident or says that parents must not find out about it. He is willing to take part in the conversation. The young person says that he has probably overdone it and wants to drink less in the future)

Counsellor: "I think it's really good that you're willing to have a conversation with me, even though I'm sure you're not doing so well today. It should not be about alcohol addiction but only about your drinking habits, possible wishes for change and how you could talk to your parents about it"

▶ Example 3

Adolescent: (tells the counsellor that he wants to drink less in the future and is glad to be able to talk to someone about support options)

Counsellor: "I think it's really good that you want to talk about yesterday's incident. We're not going to talk about alcohol addiction, but about how you can manage to drink in a more controlled way in the future. We have about 45 min to do that today"

▶ Example 4

Adolescent: (expresses to the counsellor that he would like support to deal with alcohol in a more controlled way in the future)

Counsellor: "You have expressed a desire to have support to change your approach to alcohol. I think that's really good. I'd like to spend the next 45 min with you discussing just that"

▶ Example 5

Adolescent: (tells the counsellor that he has managed to drink less alcohol for a long time. But now he has drunk too much again)

Counsellor: "I understand that you had resolved to drink less and that this did not work yesterday. I would be happy if we could talk about additional ways to successfully implement your plan. We would have about 45 min to do that today"

The counsellor points out that it is also a special situation for parents to have to collect their child from hospital under these circumstances and that he would therefore also like to have a discussion with the parents.

Counsellor: "Since it is also a special situation for parents to pick up their child from the hospital under these circumstances, we also offer talks with parents as part of our project. I would therefore like to have a conversation with you following the conversation with your son. Would you be interested in this?

4.4.2 Brief Motivational Intervention for Adolescents

The brief motivational intervention is based on motivational interviewing according to Miller and Rollnick (2002, 2013; ▶ Sect. 2.8) with regard to the basic therapeutic approach and the interview techniques used. The procedure and content are based on the six components of the brief motivational intervention according to Spirito et al. (2004; ▶ Sect. 2.11). The evidence-based components of motivational interviewing are applied by providing personal feedback on risky alcohol use, emphasising the young person's responsibility for their behaviour and possible behaviour change, sharing information and advice on low-risk alcohol use, offering and discussing different options for behaviour change, and reinforcing the young person's expectation of self-efficacy.

The brief motivational intervention with the adolescent is divided into the phases:

1. Conversation starter,
2. Interview,
3. Exploration,
4. Summarize and clarify,
5. Conclusion of the interview.

An overview of the structure and contents of the brief motivational intervention with young people is provided by the memo card "Brief Motivational Intervention Adolescents", which is used as an orientation aid during the intervention. The introductory interview part consists of the questions of the HaLT Hamburg interview (▶ Fig. 5.5). A schematic overview of the course of the intervention is given in ◘ Fig. 4.1.

Conversation Starter

Aims of the "Motivierende Kurzintervention Jugendliche" (Brief Motivational Intervention for Adolescents)

Phase: Start of conversation

- Provide an overview of the objectives of the interview
- Establishing an empathic relationship based on partnership
- Emphasis on the young person's freedom of choice and responsibility for his or her decision to change behaviour.
- Establish cooperation

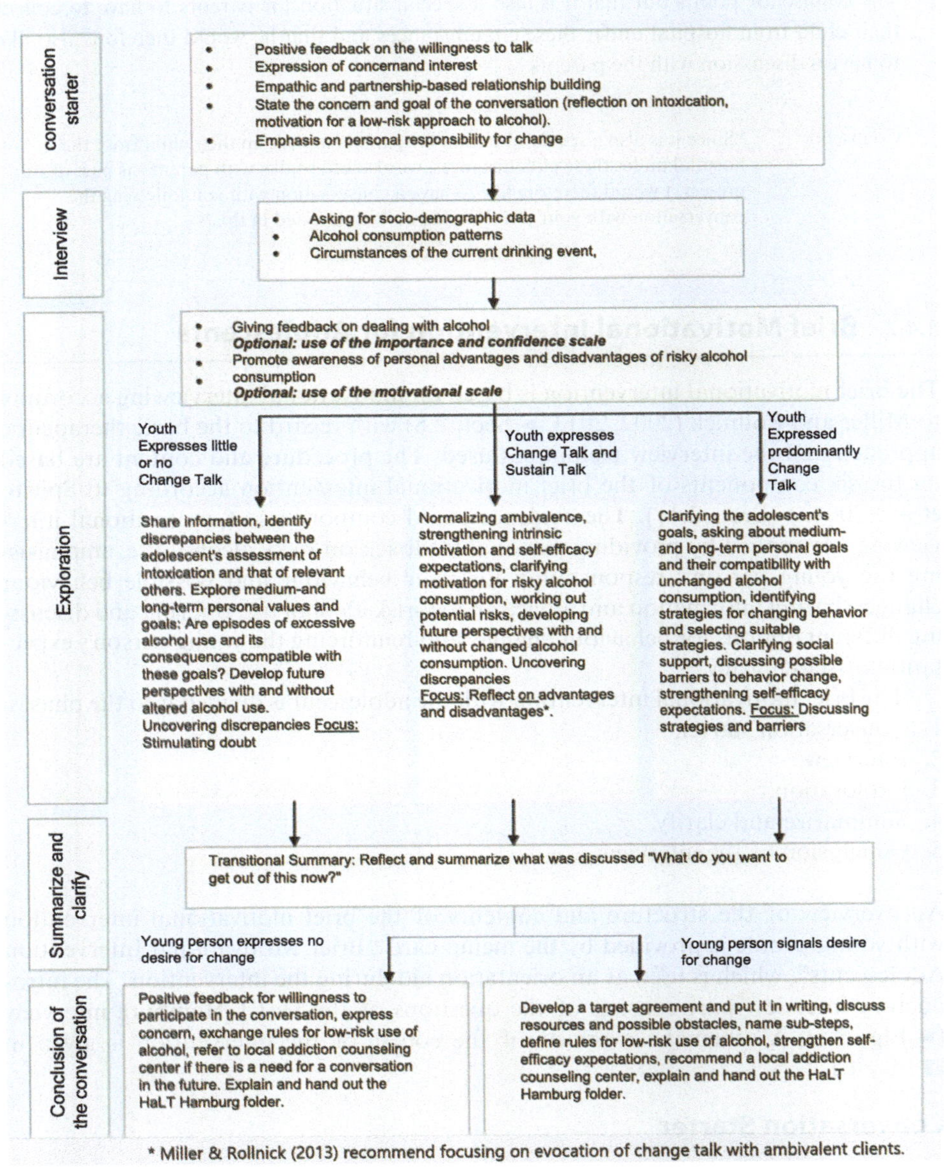

Fig. 4.1 Flow chart of the brief motivational intervention

The counsellor encourages the development of a partnership relationship between him and the young person by expressing appreciation about things that have come to his attention so far. This can be, for example, his dealings with his parents, his willingness to cooperate or his attentiveness. He or she relates his comments to the particular situation in which the young person finds himself. He or she conveys his empathetic and appreciative attitude by, among other things, demonstrating his ability to adopt the young person's perspective and, for example, formulating hypotheses about the young person's state of health (physical and psychological). The more individually he or she responds to the young person, the more authentic will be the relationship that develops in the course of the intervention. From the first contact with the young person, the counsellor therefore pays attention to behaviour and expressions that represent possible starting points for appreciation, positive reinforcement and the development of motivation to change behaviour.

Counsellor:	"Your father is very concerned about you. I have a feeling he is very upset about not being able to protect you from this experience. I find it very remarkable how calmly you responded to him"
Adolescent:	"Well, he just gets all worked up"
Counsellor:	"… and would like to persuade you to stop partying so wildly?"
Adolescent:	"Yeah, normal"
Counsellor:	"I'd like to tell you what *I*'d like to talk to you about today. Is that okay with you?"

The counsellor gives the young person an overview of the conversation to be expected and explains that he or she believes that the young person knows himself best and is therefore best placed to decide for him- or herself what is good for him or her and what is not (emphasis on freedom of choice and autonomy). This implies a great deal of freedom, but at the same time responsibility. It is not the counsellor's job to tell the young person what they can and cannot do. Alcohol intoxication is life-threatening and therefore the counsellor wants to discuss with the young person whether they are interested in learning a low-risk way of using alcohol and, if so, what this might look like. Any information the counsellor gives the young person in this conversation is an offer. The decision to use the information to change behaviour or not is up to the young person.

The counsellor will now explain that they would like to start with a few questions about the young person and the circumstances of the alcohol intoxication and will get the young person's agreement to this approach. Following the questions, there will be time for an open discussion. The counsellor emphasises that this conversation is subject to confidentiality and the contents discussed will not be passed on to parents or third parties.[4]

Counsellor:	"I'd like to start with a few questions to learn a little more about you and how the alcohol poisoning happened. Following that, I'd like to talk to you about how you'd like to deal with alcohol in the future. Is that okay with you?"

4 At the end of the discussion with the young person, you can ask separately whether the contents of the written target agreement may be communicated to the parents.

HaLT Hamburg Interview

The counsellor now starts with the HaLT Hamburg interview to collect socio-demographic data, the circumstances of alcohol intoxication and the substance history (► Fig. 5.5).

> **Aims of the "Motivierende Kurzintervention Jugendliche" (Brief Motivational Intervention for Adolescents)**
>
> **Phase: Interview**
>
> - Collect information about the person and drinking habits
> - Identify initial starting points for motivation to change
> - Giving normative feedback
> - Assess readiness for change

The counsellor familiarises him/herself with the response formats and options prior to his/her interview so that the completion of the questionnaire disrupts the interview flow as little as possible. The counsellor uses all the information from the interview part to identify possible starting points for motivation to change and to comment appreciatively on approaches to minimising the risk of alcohol consumption that have already been thought of or implemented and to take them up for the further course of the interview. Even during the entire interview section, the counsellor responds individually to the young person's answers as required. If, for example, experiences of violence or sexual assault come up, the counsellor addresses these topics flexibly before continuing with the interview questions.[5]

Exploration Phase

In this phase, the main concern is to develop ambivalence about drinking habits, i.e. to stimulate doubts in the adolescent about his or her drinking habits.

> **Aims of the "Motivierende Kurzintervention Jugendliche" (Brief Motivational Intervention for Adolescents)**
>
> **Phase: Exploration**
>
> → Develop motivation to implement a low-risk approach to alcohol, through:
>
> - Establishing rapport and building trust
> - Create awareness of personal advantages and disadvantages of risky alcohol consumption
> - Identify risks and exchange information
> - Developing future perspectives with and without altered alcohol consumption
> - Identify discrepancies between medium and long-term values and goals and the effects of excessive alcohol consumption.

---

5 Miller and Rollnick (2013) point out the so-called "assessment trap", the danger of disrupting the relationship-building process through too much diagnostics at the beginning of a conversation. However, the experiences of the counsellors in the HaLT Hamburg research project have shown that the oral interview used here has a positive effect on the course of the conversation and the relationship building.

As a transition to the exploration phase, the counsellor summarises his impression of the young person's use of alcohol (transitional summary) and gives the young person feedback by relating his personal alcohol consumption to that of his age group.

Counsellor:	"You said you drink alcohol two to three times a week, usually five or six glasses. If we compare that to the alcohol consumption of young people in your age group, 16–17 year olds, you drink significantly more than most young people your age"
Adolescent:	"What? That can't be. My friends all drink as much as I do!"
Counsellor:	"It surprises you that you drink a lot compared to your age group"
Adolescent:	"Yeah, sure. My friends all drink as much as I do, it's nothing special"
Counsellor:	"We often tend to surround ourselves with people who have similar habits and preferences to ourselves. That's why you may have the impression that you don't drink that much, even though many of your peers drink less"
Adolescent:	"That could be"

As a segue into the exploration of ambivalence about risky drinking, the counsellor may present the young person with the 'importance scale' (► Fig. 5.7).

Counsellor:	"If you were to tell me on a scale of 0–10 how important it would be to you right now to drink less, what would you say? On this scale, "0" stands for "not important at all" and "10" stands for "very important""

The counsellor can additionally present the young person with the confidence scale and ask how confident the young person would be that he or she would manage to drink alcohol in such a controlled way that he or she would no longer get drunk if he or she set his or her mind to it. Analogous to the importance scale, "0" on the confidence scale also means "not at all confident" and "10" means "completely confident." These two instruments provide the counsellor with information about the motivation to change and self-efficacy expectations regarding a change in alcohol consumption, which can be valuable starting points for the further course of the interview. Depending on how motivated the young person is to change his or her approach to alcohol or whether the young person has already developed and applied strategies to minimise the risk of his or her alcohol consumption, different emphases are set in the exploration phase.

It is important that the counsellor remains aware of his basic therapeutic stance even if the young person does not initially signal a willingness to change, and continues to work on the development of a cooperative, empathic relationship. The information the counselor conveys and the content he or she discusses with the adolescent are offers to the adolescent. The decision as to how the youth uses the information is the sole responsibility of the youth. The counsellor also emphasises this freedom of choice in the conversation with the young person in order to reduce resistance in this way[6] and to create the greatest possible openness for the topics to be discussed.

Counsellor:	*(Youth indicated a "1" on the importance scale)* "You say it is not very important to you to change your approach to alcohol. Why didn't you give a "0"?"
Adolescent:	"I might as well have ticked the '0' box"

This response indicates a low level of cooperation and resistance.[7] The counsellor avoids argumentative confrontation and applies strategies of smooth handling of resistance.[8]

Counsellor:	"What would have to happen for you to mark a "4" or a "5", for example?"
Adolescent:	"If I just couldn't handle it anymore"
Counsellor:	"How would you know?"
Adolescent:	(Thinks) "If my education were in jeopardy"

The very question of why the young person did not tick '0' offers the opportunity to trigger self-motivating statements (change talk) by reflecting on potentially detrimental aspects of alcohol consumption. It should be noted here that the vast majority of young people, when asked why a lower number on the importance scale was not selected, responded with Change Talk, unlike in the example (e.g. "Well, sometimes it's a bit much when I feel so bad after a night out partying"). Asking what would have to change or what kind of event would have to occur to increase the importance of changing one's approach to alcohol provides another opportunity for reflection on the possible consequences of risky drinking. The answers can be used as an indication of the adolescent's medium or long-term goals and can provide information about the adolescent's value system, two important starting points for promoting motivation to change.

> Two questions are particularly helpful in working with the importance scale:
> 1. "Why didn't you check "0" (or other lower number)?"
> 2. "What would have to happen for you to tick an "8" (or other higher number)?"

In response to these two open questions, the adolescent will react with change talk, i.e. he or she will give arguments why a change in behaviour is not entirely unimportant to him or her or under which circumstances the importance of a change in behav-

---

6 According to Miller and Rollnick (2013): Dissonance in the counselor-client relationship due to paternalism.

7 According to Miller and Rollnick (2013), such an utterance (sustain talk) could be an expression of nonambivalence, or it could be an expression of dissonance in the counselor-client relationship

8 Miller and Rollnick (2013) recommend in particular the use of open questions and reflective listening as well as other communication strategies (► Sect. 2.8.4).

iour would increase. Contraindicated in MI is the question "Why didn't you tick a (higher number)?". The adolescent then argues in response why a change in behaviour is not so important to him (sustain talk).

The counsellor now discusses the pros and cons of episodic excessive drinking with the young person. If the adolescent is strongly ambivalent about his excessive alcohol use, you can use the motivational scale of decision-making.[9] For this purpose, the counsellor notes down the adolescent's respective answers on the chart provided for this purpose and uses this to illustrate the ambivalence.

Counsellor:	"So your education is very important to you and you wouldn't want to put that education in jeopardy. I'd like to write that down on this sheet sometime, what we're about to discuss, so that we don't immediately forget the thoughts we have now. Is that all right with you?"
Adolescent:	"Yes"
Counsellor:	"What else could happen that would make you think about rethinking your approach to alcohol?"

The counsellor discusses the disadvantages, but also the advantages of excessive drinking for the young person. By discussing the advantages, the counsellor gets hints about the young person's motivation to drink and about the circumstances in which risky alcohol consumption occurs more often. This is important information that can be revisited as the conversation progresses and incorporated into the development of a plan of action in the form of possible barriers and impediments to controlled drinking. The motivation scale can also be used to summarise the discussed advantages and disadvantages of an unchanged or a changed approach to alcohol.

Counsellor:	"If you now look at the advantages and disadvantages of your current use of alcohol, which would outweigh the others for you at the moment? It is not only the number of advantages and disadvantages that counts, but also how important each aspect is to you"

If the adolescent mentions no or few disadvantages, the counsellor can develop hypotheses about possible disadvantages of risky alcohol consumption.

Counsellor:	"Young girls and women in particular often worry about unwanted sexual assault, which quite often happens when a girl is fully drunk and defenseless. What's it like for you?"

9 According to the latest research findings, Miller and Rollnick no longer recommend the use of the motivational scale with highly ambivalent clients, as its use triggers sustain talk as well as change talk. They recommend its use especially with clients who already have a high motivation to change, since its use with these clients mainly triggers change talk (Miller & Rose, 2015; Miller & Rollnick, 2013).

The counsellor exchanges information with the young person about various potential disadvantages of excessive alcohol consumption (see the following overviews). Wherever possible, the counsellor takes up remarks made by the young person or the parents during the previous conversation and thus shapes his hypotheses on the potential advantages and disadvantages of alcohol consumption as individually as possible. The counsellor is careful not to represent the disadvantages of alcohol use unilaterally, in order to avoid pushing the young person into the role of representing the advantages. The counsellor shows concern for the young person's use of alcohol and makes the low-risk use of alcohol clear as his or her concern, but remains true to his or her stance as a 'clarification helper'.

Risks of Episodic Excessive Alcohol Consumption for Adolescents

- Exposure in front of friends, acquaintances, possible partners
- Exposure on the Internet
- Involuntary sexual assault
- Increased risk of accidents and injuries
- Financial cost of alcohol
- Restriction of freedoms by parents
- Danger to life (e.g. through choking on vomit, freezing to death in the open)

Potential Motivations for Episodic Excessive Drinking Among Adolescents

- Group membership
- Disinhibition
- Facilitated contact (with persons of the opposite sex)
- Sensation Seeking
- Deliberate violation of the norm
- Coping strategy for dealing with negative feelings, e.g. stress, frustration

The counsellor sensitises the adolescent to the consequences of excessive drinking by generating hypotheses about possible disadvantages together with the adolescent and by reporting on what other adolescents perceive as disadvantages (see following overview). By asking circular questions, the counsellor encourages the young person to look at his or her own behaviour from different perspectives of relevant reference persons.

Counsellor:	"What would your girlfriend say if I asked her how she felt about you having alcohol poisoning today?"
Adolescent:	"Well, not so great"
Counsellor:	"What concerns might she have?"
Adolescent:	"She's just scared something's gonna happen to me or something"

Counsellor: "… What could that be?"

Adolescent: "… For example, that I get into a fight"

Counsellor: "And how do you feel about that?"

Adolescent: "Well, it's happened before"

Counsellor: "So that would be a legitimate fear?"

Motivations for Low-Risk Alcohol Consumption Among Adolescents (After Dimeff et al., 1999): What Adolescents Can Avoid and Achieve Through Low-Risk Alcohol Consumption

→ What teens can avoid:

- Having a hangover
- Exposure
- Weight gain
- Pressure from parents and school regarding grades
- Long-term health damage
- Development of tolerance

→ What young people can achieve:

- More fun due to lower blood alcohol concentration
- Financial savings
- Better school grades
- Improved control
- Reduced risk of involvement in violent acts and/or (traffic) accidents

The counsellor also asks about the adolescent's medium- and long-term personal values and goals. Are episodes of excessive alcohol consumption and their consequences compatible with these goals? Together with the young person he develops future perspectives with and without changed alcohol consumption.

Counsellor: "What would happen if you didn't change your approach to alcohol? What might your life look like in a year's time?"

Summarize and Clarify

In the preceding phases of the interview, the counsellor discussed the circumstances and background of the alcohol intoxication together with the young person. Personal drinking motivations and undesirable consequences of excessive alcohol consumption were examined and future perspectives with unchanged and low-risk drinking behaviour were developed. In the summary and clarification phase, the counsellor gives the young person another opportunity to ask questions or address issues that have not been mentioned so far, and summarises what has been discussed so far.

Aims of the "Motivierende Kurzintervention Jugendliche" (Brief Motivational Intervention for Adolescents)

Phase: Summarizing and clarifying

- Summarize and reflect on the individual advantages and disadvantages of excessive alcohol consumption.
- Strengthening intrinsic motivation for change by emphasising the young person's freedom of choice and responsibility
- Question to the young person about the personal conclusion of what has been discussed

The counsellor summarises what has been said and reflects on the advantages and disadvantages of excessive alcohol consumption mentioned by the young person, with a particular focus on highlighting the change talk expressed by the young person and relating this to the future prospects discussed. The goal of this phase of the brief motivational intervention is, if possible, the young person's decision to use alcohol in a low-risk manner. A sustainable change in behaviour can only develop from an intrinsically motivated decision. The counsellor therefore emphasises the young person's freedom of choice in this phase of the conversation as well with regard to the consequences he or she wishes to draw from what has been discussed.

Counsellor: "We've talked a lot about the role alcohol plays in your life right now. You like to drink and you just enjoy it. Drinking alcohol is part of the fun you have with your buddies and you say you can't imagine your free time without getting drunk. On the other hand, you also say that you easily get into trouble, get into fights or other trouble with the police when you have drunk a lot and that you are afraid that your residence permit might not be renewed again because of that. You had noticed that drinking a lot could be a serious problem for your goal to stay and live here in Germany in the long run. Once you look at all of this as a whole picture, what do you want to make of it?"

Conclusion of the Interview

The counsellor now works out individual drinking goals together with the young person. Together, the counsellor and the young person talk about specific frequencies and quantities, types of alcoholic beverages and situations in which controlled drinking is allowed, and situations in which the young person would like to abstain from alcohol altogether. In the process of working out the drinking goals, the counsellor offers information and advice on rules for the low-risk use of alcohol:

Messages and Information on Low-Risk Alcohol Consumption

- The effects of high-proof alcohol are difficult to assess for children and adolescents and are very harmful. I recommend that you do not drink alcohol (this recommendation always applies to children under the age of 14).
- The law for the protection of minors allows the purchase of beer and wine from the age of 16 and spirits from the age of 18. The body and especially the brain of adolescents are still developing and are more damaged by alcohol than adults. Therefore, you should start drinking alcohol as late as possible, especially high-proof alcohol.
- Do not "drink" alcohol, but drink slowly and in small sips and with breaks (e.g. one glass of alcoholic beverages, two glasses of non-alcoholic beverages). Especially with mixed drinks, keep an eye on the alcohol content, as the effect is unpredictable.
- Take into account that the blood alcohol level is at its highest only after about three quarters of an hour. The effect is therefore delayed. If you have drunk very quickly, the effect comes violently and quickly.
- Never drink alcohol in certain situations: when swimming (can be life-threatening), no moped, no bike, no car.
- Do not get into the car with a drunk driver. Make sure you know how to get home beforehand.
- No sexual intercourse when you are heavily intoxicated.
- Don't drink alone.
- Do not drink when you are sad or in a bad mood.

After setting the goals, the counsellor discusses the strategies for achieving the goals. Here, too, he is as concrete as possible, lets the young person name partial steps and considers together with the young person which resources can be used to support the intentions to act, e.g. people who can provide social support. Possible barriers and obstacles are discussed and strategies for dealing with them are developed. After discussing these topics, the young person fills in a goal agreement (▶ Fig. 5.8).

The counsellor ends the conversation with the young person by again expressing his appreciation for the willingness to talk. He encourages the young person in his self-efficacy expectations regarding the fulfilment of the discussed goals with regard to a low-risk use of alcohol.

Subsequently, the counsellor introduces a local addiction counselling centre as a possibility for further counselling. If the intervention is carried out within the framework of the project HaLT–Hart am LimiT, there is typically a cooperating addiction counselling centre that offers the so-called "risk check" especially for young people who have received a motivating brief intervention in hospital, in which young people can learn more about their own risk behaviour and their risk competences in the group. In the risk check, the young person undergoes an in-depth reflection process on his or her consumption behaviour. The aim is to learn risk competence. The central aspects of the risk check are summarised in the following overview.

Messages to Young People on the Risk Check

- You're getting info on alcohol.
- There is an exchange with other young people who have experienced the same thing.
- You can learn where your own personal boundaries are and how to take care of them.
- Taking a risk is positive, endangering yourself is reckless and life threatening.
- The offer is free of charge.
- You can bring a friend
- The risk check is a valuable opportunity—use it!

Finally, the counsellor hands out the HaLT Hamburg information folder to the young person and explains its contents and purpose. He explains that the folder contains information on how to deal with alcohol and information on a local addiction counselling centre.

If the young person does not express any wish to change his drinking behaviour after the summary of what has been discussed, the counsellor comments appreciatively on the young person's willingness to take part in the conversation. He informs the young person that he would like to give him a few rules on how to deal with alcohol in a low-risk manner. Whether he then uses these rules is up to the young person. Even in this last phase of the conversation, the counsellor should not deviate from his respectful and appreciative attitude and give in to the "correction reflex". The counsellor asks the young person for his permission to tell him the rules for low-risk use of alcohol and makes it clear that his concern is to pass this information on to the young person. How and whether he then uses the information is entirely up to him.

4.5 Parental Interview

The counsellor returns to the parents. He or she expresses his appreciation again for the parents' willingness to participate in the conversation and then presents his conversation concern. The counsellor also uses motivational interviewing techniques during the parent intervention.

Counsellor: "Alcohol poisoning is a serious matter and I am sure you are very concerned about your son. I appreciate you taking the time to speak with me anyway. Now that I have spoken with your son, I would like to discuss with you how *you feel* about your son's alcohol intoxication"

The aim of parent intervention is to provide parents or guardians with all the necessary and requested information to facilitate a supportive approach to their daughter or son. This includes information about different forms of adolescent alcohol consumption, which should enable the parents or guardians to assess whether their son is currently more likely to try alcohol, whether it is harmful use or whether there is a risk of addiction. In addition, the parental role model function in dealing with alcohol and other addictive substances such as tobacco is addressed.

Goals of the "Parent Intervention

→ Impart knowledge and develop strategies to support the adolescent in reducing the risk of alcohol consumption, by:

- Recognise: Explain indicators of risk of addiction, differences between experimental and harmful use.
- Understanding Discuss individual and adolescent causes of risky alcohol consumption. Reflect on the parents' approach to alcohol.
- Support: Clarification of whether low-risk alcohol consumption by the adolescent is an acceptable goal for behaviour modification. Discussion of strategies for achieving the goal, strengthening parental role model behaviour in dealing with addictive substances, information about techniques of motivating conversation in dealing with the son; presentation of the local addiction counselling centre.

4.5.1 Recognition

There are different types of substance use, which differ in frequency, quantity and, above all, in the effects of consumption. It is often important for parents to be able to assess what kind of alcohol consumption their child engages in and how they can therefore assess his or her risk. In distinguishing between substance use and substance misuse, the following perspectives are considered according to Newcomb and Bentler (1989) (▶ Sect. 2.6), whereby the aspects mentioned can be indicators of substance misuse either individually or in combination.

- Substance and consumption circumstances:
  - With regard to the substance consumed, a distinction is made as to how great the hazard potential of the substance is in terms of toxic, psychotropic and physiological effects.
  - Circumstances of use can serve as an indication of the distinction between substance use and abuse. Both the quantity and the duration of the period of use are assessed, as well as the appropriateness or inappropriateness of use for the situation in question.
- Person:
  - According to Newcomb and Bentler (1989), substance abuse occurs when the adolescent is unable to implement controlled use because of his or her stage of development or circumstances. Substance abuse also occurs when use interferes with age-appropriate development.
- Reaction:
  - Substance abuse is always said to occur when the adolescent's ability to function in everyday life is significantly impaired by use and signs of physical dependence can be detected.

- Consequences:
  - The consequences of consumption behaviour are also taken into account when assessing the existence of substance misuse. Here, effects of consumption on health, on social relationships and e.g. conflicts with the law are considered.

From the above-mentioned aspects, an overall picture must be drawn up in order to be able to assess the risk posed to an individual young person by his or her alcohol consumption. However, the boundaries between experimental use and harmful use are fluid.

4.5.2 Understanding

Another concern of the parent intervention is to promote the parents' willingness and ability to adopt a perspective in order to strengthen the parents' supportive approach to their son, which avoids provoking unnecessary reactance. In order to achieve this, the counsellor offers to provide the parents with information about typical adolescent motivations for alcohol consumption. An overview of developmental tasks and corresponding functions of substance use according to Silbereisen and Reese (2001) is provided in ▶ Table 2.1 (▶ Sect. 2.3). The counsellor also encourages reflection on the parents' use of alcohol by asking what experiences the parents may have had themselves in dealing with alcohol when they were at the age their son or daughter is currently.

The next step is for the counsellor to clarify whether low-risk drinking might be an acceptable goal for the parents to support their son or daughter in (for children under 14, a recommendation for abstinence is made). The counsellor presents the rules for low-risk use of alcohol, which they have also discussed with the young person, and tells the parents what intentions for behaviour change their son or daughter has shared in the previous conversation, assuming that the young person has agreed to the sharing of information. The counsellor encourages an exchange of information on how parents can support their daughter or son in learning and implementing low-risk consumption. The following overview gives suggestions on which strategies can be helpful to better implement rules in the family.

Suggestions for Parents on How to Deal with Rules

- Children need clear rules.
- Rules must be understood and comprehensible.
- Rules should be verifiable and consistently enforced.
- Quarrels often arise in families because rules are set but not followed.
- Parents should be a role model for children in dealing with rules. To this end, they should also reflect on their own use of addictive substances such as alcohol or nicotine.

The counsellor discusses with the parents what communication about conflictual issues has looked like so far and offers to provide information about ways of integrating motivational interviewing techniques into family communication. He or she shares his or her own experiences of counselling, specifically experiences of young people's reactions when confronted with pressure. The counsellor explains the approach of partnership relationship building and its benefits in terms of resistance and cooperation.

4.5.3 Support

Depending on whether the parents or guardians react to the alcohol intoxication of the adolescent in a rather overwhelmed and very concerned or rather trivialising way, the counsellor puts their responsibility for the adolescent's behaviour into perspective. For overstrained parents it is relieving to learn that they are not solely responsible for the alcohol intoxication of their son or daughter, but that with increasing age he or she becomes more and more responsible for his or her own actions and the influence of the parents becomes more and more limited:

Recommendation for Action for Concerned Parents

- Seek dialogue with the young person
- Do not pressure the young person to talk
- Create a trusting and calm atmosphere
- Select a suitable time and place
- Addressing parental concerns openly
- Avoiding accusations, insinuations and threats
- Take a clear position

On the other hand, parents of underage children have a duty of care and are obliged to protect their child from behaviour that is harmful to themselves and others, which should be emphasised especially in the case of parents who trivialise the situation:

Rules for Low-Risk Handling of Alcohol for Parents

- Make parents aware of their own consumption and the possible connection with consumption patterns of their children → Role model function ("How do you deal with alcohol in the family?")
- The issue of supervision as an important topic, especially for younger adolescents
- Parents should be informed and should also pass on this information to their children (so that young people understand why rules are agreed)
- Talk about rules together: low-risk consumption at the party, how and when the daughter or son will come home, who will accompany them to the party; possible consequences if alcohol is consumed excessively again despite agreed rules.
- Parents can get further information and support → local addiction counselling centre, counselling also provided by other institutions when it comes to topics concerning further educational issues or health aspects (e.g. general social service, counselling centres for sexualised/domestic violence, specialist doctors)

The counsellor records the goals formulated together with the parents in writing in the goal agreement. Together, the necessary partial steps and social support are named as concretely as possible. The parents draw up the target agreement and receive information about the counselling services offered by the local addiction counselling centre.

4.6 Final Discussion

For the final interview, the counsellor meets again with the guardians and the young person. This part of the conversation should be kept as short as possible in order not to impair the effects of the individual interventions. The aim of the final discussion is to strengthen the self-efficacy expectations of the adolescent and the parents with regard to their expressed intentions to change behaviour and to positively reinforce their willingness to talk and to deal with the issue of alcohol consumption.

Objectives of the "Final Discussion"

→ Strengthening self-efficacy expectations, appreciation, outlook

- Express appreciation for expressed intentions to change behavior.
- Summarise agreed strategies of parents and young person (if permission is given)
- Phone booster outlook
- Strengthen self-efficacy expectations

Provided the counsellor has obtained the young person's consent to communicate their behaviour change goals and strategies agreed during the intervention, the counsellor again summarises the agreed risk reduction goals and strategies for the young person and the agreed support strategies for the parents and expresses their appreciation of the decisions made.

Counsellor: *(to the teenager)* "I think it's really great that you were willing to have this conversation with me here in the hospital. Not only that, but I get the feeling that it's really really important to you that you don't want to drink yourself into unconsciousness again, and you've had a whole lot of good ideas about how to make sure you do that from now on. Do you want to tell your parents about what you agreed with me earlier?"

The counsellor involves the parents in the conversation and explains the agreed role of the parents in supporting the son to achieve the alcohol use goals he has set.

Counsellor: *(to the parents)* "You said in our conversation that you want to support your son in this and that you would like to sit down with him again at home to find out more about what your son does in his free time and with whom. You also said that you don't want to blame, you just want to understand more so you can be more supportive. *(Parent agrees)*. *(to the teenager)* What do you think?"

The counsellor mediates between parents and adolescent and provides as positive a basis as possible for further support of the adolescent by the parents, on which further communication can take place after discharge from hospital. If necessary, the counsellor again recommends a visit to the local addiction counselling centre for further counselling and assistance or the risk check. If there are specific issues relating to parenting or physical/mental health, the counsellor will refer the young patient to further help. The counsellor bids farewell to the parents and the young person with an encouraging, self-efficacy-promoting comment.

4.7 HaLT-Hamburg Discussion Documentation

At the end of the interview with the young person and the guardians, the counsellor documents the conversation. He checks whether all the information in the HaLT Hamburg interview has been answered completely and, if necessary, completes any missing information according to the adolescent's oral statements in the interview. The interview documentation sheet is also filled out after the interviews with the young person and the parents have been completed. In the interview documentation, among other things, the manual adherence is recorded and an assessment of the readiness for change, the framework conditions of the intervention as well as possible psychological comorbidities (suspected diagnosis) is given. The data from the interview documentation and the HaLT Hamburg interview can be used for the following purposes:

1. Evaluate conditions of sustainable implementation, ensure long-term quality monitoring, and
2. Developments and trends in risky alcohol consumption in the to capture the risk population of underage binge drinkers.

Materials and Further Literature

Contents

S. Diestelkamp, R. Thomasius, *Risky Alcohol Consumption among Adolescents*,
https://doi.org/10.1007/978-3-662-68635-5_5

5.1 Materials for the Implementation of the Intervention

On the following pages you will find the materials for conducting the intervention as copy templates. These are:

- Memo card Welcome and introduction of the project, ▫ Fig. 5.1
- Memo card Brief Motivational Intervention Adolescents, ▫ Fig. 5.2
- Memo Card Parent Intervention, ▫ Fig. 5.3
- Memo card Final Discussion, ▫ Fig. 5.4
- HaLT Hamburg Interview, ▫ Fig. 5.5
- Motivation Scale template, ▫ Fig. 5.6
- Importance and Confidence Scale template, ▫ Fig. 5.7
- Template goal agreement adolescents, ▫ Fig. 5.8
- Template goal agreement parents, ▫ Fig. 5.9
- Interview documentation for counsellors, ▫ Fig. 5.10
- Telephone booster guide, ▫ Fig. 5.11
- Template Information Sheet, ▫ Fig. 5.12

HaLT-Hamburg

HaLT-Hamburg

Memo card welcome and introduction of the project

- Presentation person and function
- Appreciation for the willingness to talk
- Naming the concern:
  - ☐ More and more young people have to be treated for alcohol poisoning in Hamburg clinics
  - ☐ HaLT-Hamburg as a project to reduce risky alcohol consumption among young people
  - ☐ Content: Interview with young person and parents and survey
  - ☐ Goal: Risk competence in dealing with alcohol and reflection on what has happened.
  - ☐ Duration: each conversation about half an hour

- Question about interest in participation -> more detailed information on:
  - ☐ Procedure of the talks in the clinic
  - ☐ Data protection and confidentiality

- Handing out the consent form
  - ☐ Explanation of questions
  - ☐ Signature

Fig. 5.1 Memo card welcoming and introducing the project

HaLT-Hamburg

HaLT-Hamburg

Memo Card Motivating Brief Intervention Adolescents

Conversation starter

- ☐ Positive feedback on the willingness to talk
- ☐ Expression of concern and interest
- ☐ Empathic and partnership relationship offer
- ☐ State the concern and goal of the conversation:
  → Reflection of what has happened and risk competence in dealing with alcohol.
- ☐ Emphasis on personal responsibility for change
- ☐ Provide an overview of the process:
  → Start with questions about the person and the drinking habits and circumstances (interview) and then open discussion part.

Interview

- ☐ Conducting the HaLT Hamburg interview

Exploration

- ☐ Provide feedback on drinking habits
- ☐ Background and motivation of excessive alcohol consumption
- ☐ *Optional: use of the importance and confidence scale*
- ☐ Advantages and disadvantages of risky use of alcohol
  → *Optional: use of the motivational scale*
  → Stimulate ideas about advantages and disadvantages by:
    - circular questioning
    - Give information
- ☐ Development of future perspectives with changed and unchanged alcohol consumption

→ Clarification of medium- and long-term goals and compatibility with excessive alcohol consumption.

Summarize and clarify

- ☐ Reflect and summarize advantages and disadvantages of unchanged alcohol consumption
- ☐ "What would you like to make of it now?"

Conclusion of the conversation

- ☐ Development of strategies for consumption and risk management
- ☐ Develop drinking goals
- ☐ Discuss possible barriers
- ☐ Clarification of resources
- ☐ Fill out target agreement

- ☐ Appreciation of the willingness to talk
- ☐ Strengthen self-efficacy expectations
- ☐ Presentation of Kö16A
- ☐ Info about participation in the risk check
- ☐ Handing out the HaLT Hamburg information folder

Fig. 5.2 Memo card Brief Motivational Intervention Adolescents

HaLT-Hamburg

HaLT-Hamburg

Memo Card Parent Intervention

Introduction

- ☐ Appreciation with regard to the willingness to talk
- ☐ Presentation of the discussion concern:
  → Offer to talk to clarify questions
  → Provide suggestions for dealing with the situation and helping the adolescent avoid future alcohol intoxications.
- ☐ Question about the evaluation of alcohol intoxication by the parents

Recognize

- ☐ Sharing information on indicators of probationary use / harmful use / risk of addiction.

Understand

- ☐ Discuss adolescent typical motivations for alcohol consumption.
- ☐ Reflection on parental use of alcohol and any early experiences with alcohol.

Support

- ☐ Discuss strategies to support the youth
- ☐ Rules for the low-risk use of alcohol
- ☐ Feedback on the youth's intended risk reduction strategies (if consent obtained).
- ☐ Dealing with conflicts
- ☐ Sensitization for one's own handling of addictive substances, perception of the role model function with regard to one's own consumption
- ☐ Make target agreement and write it down
- ☐ Presentation of the local addiction counseling center and recommendation to contact it
- ☐ Handing out the information folder for parents and explaining the contents

Fig. 5.3 Memo card Parent Intervention

HaLT-Hamburg

HaLT-Hamburg

Memo card final meeting

→ Strengthening self-efficacy expectations, appreciation, outlook

- ☐ Express appreciation for expressed intentions to change behavior
- ☐ Summarize agreed-upon strategies of parent and youth (if permission is granted).
- ☐ Outlook on possible contact with a local addiction counseling center
- ☐ Sign sheet for billing with health insurance companies
- ☐ Strengthen self-efficacy expectations

Fig. 5.4 Memo card Final Discussion

Hamburg

University Hospital Hamburg-Eppendorf

erman Center for Addiction Issues in Childhood and Adolescence (DZSKJ)

Client code:

Consultant initials | Day | Month | Year | Case no. today

HaLT-Hamburg Interview

(Interview for use during motivational brief bedside intervention).

HaLT-Hamburg

Authority for Health and Consumer Protection (BGV) Department of Drugs and Addiction (Head: Dr. S. Bever)

Kö16a Addiction counseling for children, Youths and Ang ependents (Direction: W. Raulf)

University Medical Center Hamburg-Eppendorf German Center for Addiction Issues of Childhood and Adolescence (DZSKJ) (Medical Director: Prof. Dr. R. Thomasius)

Fig. 5.5 HaLT Hamburg Interview

☒ **The interview must be conducted orally and completed during the interview!**

May I ask briefly in advance how old you are?

Age: ________ Years

1. **If you think about yesterday: Where did you drink?**

☐ (1) at home (without parental supervision)
☐ (2) in the home of friends (without parental supervision).
☐ (3) in a discotheque/restaurant
☐ (4) on the road/outside
☐ (5) public event (cathedral, soccer, pop/rock concert or similar)

2. **Have you been drinking with others?**

☐ (1) yes (together with other, ***additional*** ______________ persons)
☐ (0) no (alone without peers, siblings or similar)

3. **When did you start drinking? Time: ________________________ Clock**

4. **What have you been drinking?**

☐ (1) Beer
☐ (2) Wine/sparkling wine
☐ (3) Mixed drinks with spirits
☐ (4) Spirits
☐ (5) Mixed beer drinks
☐ (6) Alcopops

5. **How many of the drinks did you drink?**
Please refer to the conversion chart below! [Source: ESPAD study]

Drink	**Quanti ty**
Beer	
Wine/champagne	
Mix with spirits	
Spirits	
Mixed beer drinks	
Alcopops	

Fig. 5.5 (continued)

Please note the respective bottle and glass sizes and try to convert to "drinks"! (e.g. 1 big glass of wine = 2 drinks, 2 big beers â 0,5l = 3 drinks etc.)

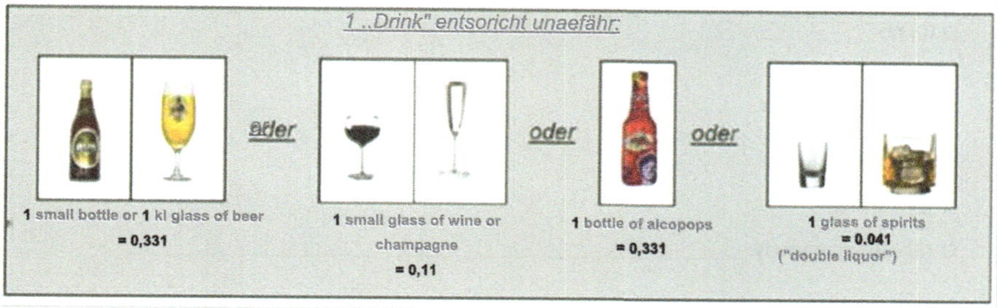

6. where was the Alko hol purchased?

a) Party or with friends (indoors)

☐ (1) self brought from home

☐ (2) self brought from the supermarket

☐ (3) self brought from the gas station

☐ (4) self brought from the kiosk / station kiosk

☐ (5) brought by yourself / **Other: .** ____________________

☐ (6) do not know / was "already there

b) Clique on the road or outside

☐ (1) self brought from home

☐ (2) self brought from the supermarket

☐ (3) self brought from the gas station

☐ (4) self brought from the kiosk / station kiosk

☐ (5) brought by yourself or **other:** ____________________

☐ (6) do not know or was "already there

c) Discotheque/restaurant

☐ (1) bought **there** itself

☐ (2) From friends

☐ (3) "donated" by other persons

d) public event/event

☐ (1) bought **there** itself

☐ (2) From friends

☐ (3) "donated" by others

Fig. 5.5 (continued)

7. Have you consumed other stimulants besides alcohol (nicotine, cannabis, etc.)?

- ☐ (1) yes
- ☐ (0) no

8. If so, which ones?

- ☐ (1) Nicotine
- ☐ (2) Cannabis
- ☐ (3) others, namely: ____________________

9. What were de.n other people mainly drinking?

WHO.	WHAT? (beer, champagne, vodka, ...)	HOW MUCH? (glasses, bottles, ...)	EFFECT?
Male adolescents ("boys")			☐ tipsy ☐ drunk ☐ full drunk
Female teenagers ("girls")			☐ tipsy ☐ drunk ☐ full drunk

10. Where were you found before you were taken to the hospital?

- ☐ (1) at home (without parental supervision)
- ☐ (2) In the home of friends (without parental supervision).
- ☐ (3) in **front of** the discotheque/restaurant/event
- ☐ (4) **in** the discotheque/restaurant/event
- ☐ (5) in the park, bushes, cellar entrance, house entrance or similar (outside)
- ☐ (6) in a strange apartment (indoors)

Exact location (street or district): ....

11. Is the whereabouts identical to the last remembered whereabouts?

- ☐ (1) not identical
- ☐ (2) Reminder correct

Fig. 5.5 (continued)

12. How were you brought in?

- ☐ (1) Ambulance (RTW)
- ☐ (2) Friends/family
- ☐ (3) Police
- ☐ (4) Other: ______________________________

13. How well can you remember yesterday?

- ☐ (1) hardly at anything
- ☐ (2) to some yes, to some no
- ☐ (3) to most

14. Do you have any injuries?

- ☐ (1) yes, ______________________________
  - Reason for injury:
    - ☐ (11) brawl
    - ☐ (12) Bicycle accident
    - ☐ (13) Car accident
    - ☐ (14) sexual assault
    - ☐ (15) Other: ______________
- ☐ (0) no

15. Have you been hospitalized before because you had too much to drink?

- ☐ (1) yes ________ Mal
- ☐ (0) no

16. If so, how many of these in the last 12 months? ______ Times

16. a) If yes, how often did you talk to a HaLT counselor? ______________ Times

17. Please think about the <u>last 30 days</u>: How often (if at all) have you had <u>5 (for girls 4!)</u> or more alcoholic drinks on one occasion? *(Please note the respective bottles and glass sizes, see conversion chart above).*

- ☐ (1) yesterday for the first time
- ☐ (2) ___ Mal and yesterday

Fig. 5.5 (continued)

CRAFFT

1. **Have you ever ridden in a car with someone who had been drinking alcohol?**

☐ (1) yes

☐ (0) no

2. **Do you drink to relax, feel better, or to feel more comfortable among friends or acquaintances?**

☐ (1) yes

☐ (0) no

3. **Do you drink alcohol when you are alone?**

☐ (1) yes

☐ (0) no

4. **Have family members or friends ever advised you to drink less?**

☐ (1) yes

☐ (0) no

5. **Have you ever forgotten something you did when you were drinking alcohol?**

☐ (1) yes

☐ (0) no

6. **Have you ever gotten in trouble with other people when you drank alcohol?**

☐ (1) yes

☐ (0) no

Fig. 5.5 (continued)

Motivation scale

HaLT-Hamburg

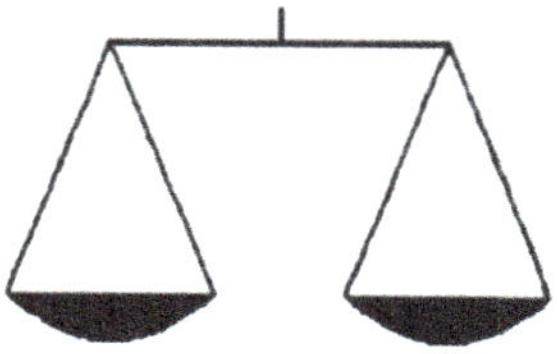

	Maintaining contact with alcohol	Changing the way we deal with alcohol
Advantages		
Disadvantages		

Fig. 5.6 Motivation Scale template

5

HaLT-Hamburg

Importance scale and confidence scale

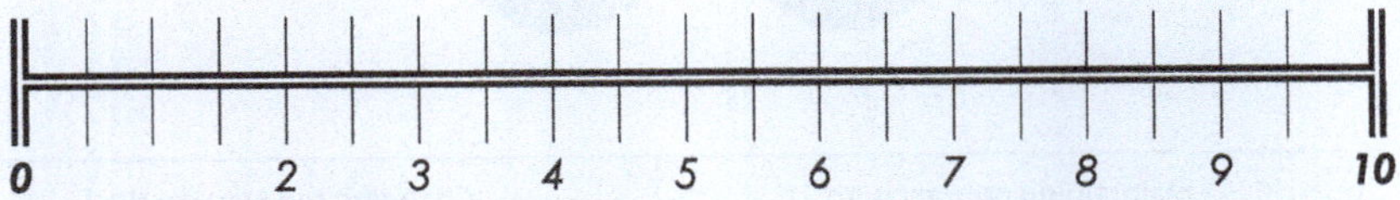

Fig. 5.7 Importance and Confidence Scale template

Target agreement

HaLT-Hamburg

________________________________ has developed the following goals and agreements at ____________ to avoid risky alcohol consumption in the future:

The following goals were formulated:

1. ____

2. ____

3. ____

The following agreements were reached:

1. ____

2. ____

3. ____

Hamburg, the ____________________

____________________ ____________________

Signature of the adolescentSignature of the counselor

Fig. 5.8 Template goal agreement youths

Target agreement parents

HaLT-Hamburg

Within the framework of the parents' meeting on __ the following goals and agreements were worked out in order to avoid risky alcohol consumption in the future by ____________ avoid:

The following goals were formulated:

1. ____________________

2. ____________________

3. ____________________

The following agreements were reached:

1. ____________________

2. ____________________

3. ____________________

Hamburg, the ____________________

____________________ ____________________

Signature of parent/guardianSignature of advisor

Fig. 5.9 Template goal agreement parents

Hamburg

University Hospital
Hamburg-Eppendorf

German Center for Addiction Issues in Childhood and Adolescence (DZSKJ)

Client code:

Consultant	Day	Month	Year	Case no.

HaLT-Hamburg
Interview documentation

(Questionnaire for counselors following the intervention).

HaLT-Hamburg

Authority for Health and Consumer Protection (BGV) Department of Drugs and Addiction (Head: Dr. S. Bever)

Kö16a Addiction counseling for children, Adolescents and relatives (Direction: W. Raulf)

University Medical Center Hamburg-Eppendorf German Center for Addiction Issues of Childhood and Adolescence (DZSKJ) (Medical Director: Prof. Dr. R. Thomasius)

Fig. 5.10 Interview documentation for counsellors

5

I. Sociodemographics

As a HaLT-HH counselor, you have learned some (or all) of the following information from your conversation with the youth and parents. *Please answer any questions about which you have received information.*

1	**Age of the young person(s)?**	________ Years	2	**Gender**	Young ☐ (1)	Girls ☐ (2)

3	**Born in which country?** ☐ (1) in Germany or ☐ (2) other country, namely ________________
5	**In which country were the parents born? Mother:** ☐ (1) in Germany or ☐ (2) other country, namely ________________ **Father:** ☐ (1) in Germany or ☐ (2) other country, namely ________________
6	**Does the young person still go to school?** (except vocational school) ☐ (1) yes ☐ (0) no, then please continue with **question 9.**
7	**Which school?** ☐ (1) Special school / special school (e.g. learning and physically handicapped school) ☐ (2) Secondary / elementary school ☐ (3) Secondary school ☐ (4) Comprehensive school / district school ☐ (5) Technical secondary school ☐ (6) High school ☐ (7) another school, namely ________________
8	**In which class?** To the ____ Class. Please continue with **question 11.**
9	**If no longer in school ... What high school diploma was obtained?** School type ________________ Grade level ________________
10	**Current activity?** ☐ (1) Training ☐ (2) Work ☐ (3) Internship ☐ (4) Free social/ecological training year. ☐ (5) unemployed ☐ (6) something completely different, namely ________________
11	**Main place of residence?** ☐ (1) for natural parents ☐ (2) for mother and her partner ☐ (3) with father and his partner ☐ (4) for mother ☐ (5) with father ☐ (6) with grandparents or other relatives ☐ (7) for foster parents/adoptive parents ☐ (8) in own apartment ☐ (9) in a home
15	Residence of the young person(s)?________________

Fig. 5.10 (continued)

I. Framework

11. **How long did the interview with the adolescent last?**

Time required: approx. ___ Minutes

12. **How long did the conversation with the parents last?**

Time required: approx. ___ Minutes

13. **In what setting did the interview with the youth take place?**

- ☐ (1) alone in a separate room
- ☐ (2) alone in the hospital room
- ☐ (3) In the patient room with other patients present.
- ☐ (4) In the sick room with parents present.
- ☐ (5) In a semi-public space (waiting room, hallway, lounge).
- ☐ (6) Other: ____

14. **Were there any interruptions due to external factors?**

- ☐ (1) yes
- ☐ (2) no

4.a. If yes, how many interruptions? ______________

4.b Which? ____

4.c How disruptive were the interruptions to the flow of the conversation?

- ☐ (1) not disturbing at all
- ☐ (2) little disturbing
- ☐ (3) disturbing
- ☐ (4) Very disturbing

15. **Did the adolescent express dissatisfaction with the care provided by hospital staff without being asked?**

- ☐ (1) yes
- ☐ (2) no

II. Conversation content

16. **Which topics were discussed with the young person?**

- ☐ (1) Feedback on the adolescent's drinking habits.
- ☐ (2) Background and motivation of risky alcohol consumption
- ☐ (3) Advantages and disadvantages of risky alcohol consumption
- ☐ (4) current life satisfaction
- ☐ (5) Future perspectives with and without altered alcohol consumption
- ☐ (6) Messages/risk information on alcohol consumption.

Fig. 5.10 (continued)

- ☐ (7) Consumption and risk management strategies.
- ☐ (8) Development of drinking goals
- ☐ (9) Identification of the barriers
- ☐ (10) Clarification of resources
- ☐ (11) Documentation of goals and agreements
- ☐ (12) previous use of assistance
- ☐ (13) Presentation of Kö16a
- ☐ (14) Information on participation in the risk check
- ☐ (15) Other: ____________________

III. Conversation techniques

17. Which methods of motivational interviewing were used?
(Please underline the applicable frequency!)

- ☐ (1) Express empathy .... *rarely / sometimes / often*
- ☐ (2) active listening .... *rarely / sometimes / often*
- ☐ (3) ask open questions .... *rarely / sometimes / often*
- ☐ (4) Develop discrepancy .... *rarely / sometimes / often*
- ☐ (5) Express appreciation .... *rarely / sometimes / often*
- ☐ (6) Summaries .... *rarely / sometimes / often*
- ☐ (7) go with the resistance .... *rarely / sometimes / often*
- ☐ (8) Strengthen self-efficacy .... *rarely / sometimes / often*

18. Which instruments were used?

- ☐ (1) Importance scale
- ☐ (2) Confidence scale
- ☐ (3) 4-field scheme (motivational scale)

IV. Readiness for change

19. How do you assess the adolescent's readiness to change after the interview? The adolescent ...

- ☐ (1) drinks alcohol and does not want to change it
- ☐ (2) has thought about drinking less
- ☐ (3) Has firmly decided to drink less alcohol

V. Psychological comorbidity

20. What mental health comorbid disorders according to ICD-10 would you suspect are diagnoses?

- ☐ (F0) organic, including symptomatic mental disorders.
- ☐ (F1) mental and behavioral disorders caused by psychotropic substances.
- ☐ (F2) Schizophrenia, schizotypal and delusional disorders.

Fig. 5.10 (continued)

- ☐ (F3) affective disorders
- ☐ (F4) neurotic, stress, and somatoform disorders.
- ☐ (F5) behavioral problems with physical disorders or factors.
- ☐ (F6) Personality and behavioral disorders
- ☐ (F7) Intelligence impairment
- ☐ (F8) Developmental disorders
- ☐ (F9) Behavioral and emotional disorders with onset in childhood and adolescence.
- ☐ (FX) no suspected diagnosis

11. There was also a suspicion of ...

- ☐ (1) Child welfare endangerment
- ☐ (2) sexual abuse associated with alcohol intoxication.
- ☐ (3) Other, namely ______________________________

12. Continuing Treatment: The adolescent ...

- ☐ (1) was conveyed to Kö16a
- ☐ (2) was referred to the drug outpatient clinic of the UKE
- ☐ (3) received the flyer of the Rechtsmed. Examination center for victims of violence at the UKE
- ☐ (4) was admitted to psychiatric treatment as an inpatient
- ☐ (5) Is already receiving outpatient psychiatric/psychological treatment and will continue to do so.
- ☐ (6) Other, namely ______________________________

VI. parent interview

13. Did a discussion take place with the parents or guardians of the adolescent(s)?

- ☐ (1) yes
- ☐ (2) no

13. a) If not, reason:

- ☐ (1) no sufficient knowledge of German
- ☐ (2) No interest
- ☐ (3) Parents not present
- ☐ (4) Other, namely ______________________________

General remarks

____

____

____

____

____

____

Thank you for your cooperation!

Fig. 5.10 (continued)

Hamburg

University Hospital
Hamburg-Eppendorf

German Center for Addiction Issues in Childhood and Adolescence (DZSKJ)

Client code:

Consultant-	Day	Month	Year	Case no.

HaLT-Hamburg

Interview guide

for the

PHONE BOOSTER

HaLT-Hamburg

University Medical Center Hamburg-
Eppendorf German Center for Addiction
Issues
of Childhood and Adolescence (DZSKJ)
(Medical Director: Prof. Dr. med. R. Thomasius)

Fig. 5.11 Telephone booster guide

Preliminary remarks

The telephone booster will be conducted with the adolescents in the intervention group 6 weeks after each motivational brief intervention in the hospital. In each case, the adolescents are called by the student assistants who conducted the interview in the hospital.

Phone booster goals

- ☐ Reminder of the conversation in the hospital and the study
- ☐ **Asking about success in meeting drinking goals outlined in the goal agreement and refreshing motivation to pursue goals**
- ☐ Question about contacting the local addiction counseling center (Kö16a) or other help offers (counseling, therapy) and, if interested, passing on contact data if necessary

Preparations

In preparation for the telephone booster, the student assistant reads through the interview documentation she has prepared for this young person, paying particular attention to the following points:

- ☐ Was the young person addressed as "you" or "you"?
- ☐ Did a topic come up during the interview with the young person that could be referred to in the telephone booster? (e.g., school situation, family situation, home, leisure time, health).
- ☐ Provide information on the local addiction counseling center (address, phone number, opening hours, services offered, etc.)
- ☐ Have call documentation ready for telephone booster.

Procedure

I Conversation starter

- ☐ Presentation of the own person
  "Hello (name of young person), this is (name of student assistant), I am a staff member in the project "HaLT-Hamburg". We met 6 weeks ago at (name of clinic) where I conducted a survey with you."

II Main part

- ☐ Ask if the young person has time right now and can talk without being disturbed
  "Do you have a few minutes right now so we can talk in peace?"
- ☐ Name concerns
  "I wanted to ask how you are doing now ... "
- ☐ Let the young person report freely and ask follow-up questions. If only a short answer is given, follow up with a next question:
  "I'm glad you're doing well. Has it always been like this in the past weeks?"
  "What was it about when you were in a bad mood?
  "Have you been able to talk to anyone about it?"
  "What did you do when there was no one to talk to at the time?"

Fig. 5.11 (continued)

5

- ☐ Additional questions on topics that emerged from the hospital interview:
  " Have you been back to Flensburg in the meantime to visit the friends you have there? How was the reunion?"
  "How was your last handball tournament?"
  "It's always reported that students in tenth grade have so much on their plate, how do you create spaces for yourself?"

- ☐ **Question about the goals formulated in the conversation with the consultants and success in their implementation.**
  "During your conversation with the counselor at the hospital, had you set goals for managing alcohol?"
  "You did discuss some things in the conversation with the counselor at the hospital about how you want to deal with alcohol in the future so you don't end up in the hospital again. How has that worked out over the last few weeks?"

Goals according to the consultant's documentation	Targets mentioned during the phone booster	Assessment of the course (from the young person's point of view)	Motivation to achieve goals
1	1	1	1 ....
2	2	2	2 ....
3	3	3	3 ....

- ☐ **Reconstruction of the situations in which the achievement of the goal was successful and those in which it was not. Follow-up questions.**
  "What helped you realize your drinking goals?"
  "In what situations could you not stick to it?"
  "For what reasons did you find it difficult to stick to it?"

- ☐ Question about contacting the local counseling center or interest in contacting the local counseling center, if applicable.
  "Do you know Kö l 6a?"

Fig. 5.11 (continued)

☐ Question about seeking counseling or therapy services.
"Have you contacted any other counseling services since your hospitalization?"

☐ If needed, introduction to local counseling center. (The adolescent may not remember that she was already introduced to him at the clinic).
"If you are interested, I can give you the contact information".

III Conclusion of the phone call

☐ Appreciative and self-efficacy-enhancing closing commentary.
"I think it's great that you are now making sure that your "shuffles" are not so strong. I continue to wish you all the best with that!"
"Do you have any questions for me about the counseling center or any other topic?"
"Okay, then I thank you for your willingness and have a nice day".

IV Interview documentation

1. How long did the phone call with the teenager last?
Time required: approx. ____ Minutes

2. What environment was the youth in during the phone call?
(Interviewer's assessment)
☐ (1) alone, the adolescent could speak undisturbed
☐ (2) Alone, in public space (e.g., street, subway, supermarket).
☐ (3) With friends/acquaintances present.
☐ (4) with family members present
☐ (6) Other: ____________________

3. Were there any interruptions due to external factors?
☐ (1) yes
☐ (2) no

3.a If so, how many interruptions? ____________
3.b Which? ____________________
3.c How disruptive were the interruptions to the flow of the conversation?
☐ (1) not disturbing at all
☐ (2) little disturbing
☐ (3) disturbing
☐ (4) Very disturbing

Fig. 5.11 (continued)

II. Conversation content

4. Which complexes of topics received attention in the conversation with the young person?

☐ (1) Designation of the goals formulated with the consultant in the hospital.

→ Did the adolescent remember the goals agreed upon in the hospital?

☐ (2) yes, to all (number:__________)

☐ (3) yes, but not to all (number: __________)

☐ (4) no

☐ (5) Assessment of the achievement of the goals formulated in the hospital (progression).

☐ (6) Discussing the youth's motivation to achieve the goal.

☐ (7) inhibiting and promoting conditions of goal achievement

☐ (8) Question about utilization of a therapy or counseling service.

→ Has the adolescent taken advantage of any counseling or therapy services since hospitalization?

☐ (9) yes, namely ______________________________

☐ (10) no

☐ (11) Presentation of the local addiction counseling center.

☐ (12) Information on participation in the risk check

☐ (13) Outlook for telephone catamneses and compensation of expenses

☐ (14) Other: ______________________________

5. Through what expressions did you try to support the adolescent's motivation to achieve the goal?

☐ (1) Praise and recognition for attempts to achieve goals.

☐ (2) Expression of understanding of difficulties

☐ (3) Strengthening confidence in future attempts to achieve goals.

☐ (4) good wishes for the future

☐ (5) Formulation of an optimistic closing formula

☐ (6) Other: ______________________________

III. Conversational atmosphere

6. Did the adolescent remember being interviewed by you at the hospital?

☐ (1) yes, immediately

☐ (2) no, only after explanation

Fig. 5.11 (continued)

7. was the young person willing to talk?

- ☐ (1) yes, very willing to talk
- ☐ (2) partly, partly
- ☐ (3) no, rather taciturn
- ☐ (4) no, the adolescent dropped the phone call
  Reason: ______________________________

General remarks

____

____

____

____

____

____

Thank you for your cooperation!

Fig. 5.11 (continued)

Leaflet deployment information

HaLT-Hamburg

Phone info:

- ☐ Call at 7.00
- ☐ Introduce person and function
- ☐ Request info:
    - o Are there alcohol-intoxicated youth on site?
    - o Dude?
    - o Health insurance?
    - o Physical condition?
    - o If applicable, whether and when parents come to the hospital
- ☐ Inaccessibles: were there youth who were treated that night and have already been discharged?
    - o If yes, note reason for unavailability

Deployment information hospitals

Upon arrival :

- ☐ Ask for full name of the teenager
- ☐ Request room number
- ☐ Ask for HaLT information folder or have it at hand

Name of the clinic:	**Station:** **Phone:** **Additional station, if applicable: Phone:** **Space for conversation: Special features or to be noted:**	**Address:**
Name of the clinic:	**Station:** **Phone:** **Additional station, if applicable: Phone:** **Space for conversation: Special features or to be noted:**	**Address:**

Fig. 5.12 Template for information sheet on use

Name of the clinic:	**Station:** **Phone:** **Additional station, if applicable: Phone:** **Space for conversation: Special features or to be noted:**	**Address:**
Name of the clinic:	**Station:** **Phone:** **Additional station, if applicable: Phone:** **Space for conversation: Special features or to be noted:**	**Address:**

Fig. 5.12 (continued)

Further Reading

Diestelkamp, S., Arnaud, N., & Thomasius, R. (2014). Alcohol in childhood and adolescence—Epidemiology, early detection and treatment of harmful consumption patterns. *Pediatrics up2date, 09*(01), 15–37. https://doi.org/10.1055/s-0033-1358885

Kuhn, S., Trenkler, F., & Kalke, J. (2011). *Recommendations for parents in dealing with their children's alcohol consumption: Scientific knowledge. A guidebook for addiction prevention professionals.* Federal Ministry of Health.

Miller, W. R., & Rollnick, S. (2015). *Motivational interviewing* (3rd ed.). Lambertus.

Thomasius, R., Häßler, F., & Nesseler, T. (2009). *When adolescents drink: Ways out of flat rate drinking and coma binge drinking: Adolescents, experts and parents report.* Trias.

Supplementary Information

S. Diestelkamp, R. Thomasius, *Risky Alcohol Consumption among Adolescents*,
https://doi.org/10.1007/978-3-662-68635-5

Literature

Ajzen, I. (1985). From intentions to actions: A theory of planned behavior. In J. Kuhl & J. Beckman (Eds.), *Action control from cognition to behavior* (pp. 11–39). Springer.

Ajzen, I. (1991). The theory of planned behavior. *Organizational Behavior and Human Decision Processes, 50*, 179–211.

Armitage, C. J., & Conner, M. (2001). Efficacy of the theory of planned behavior: A meta-analytic review. *British Journal of Social Psychology, 40*(4), 471–499.

Arnaud, N., Diestelkamp, S., Wartberg, L., Sack, P.-M., Lammers, K., Kammerahl, S., & Thomasius, R. (2015). Nachhaltiger Transfer des Gesundheitsnetz Alkohol im Jugendalter: Eine Kooperation aus Forschung, Praxis und Politik. *Psychiatrische Praxis, 42*(S01), 35–38.

Baumeister, R. F., & Vohs, K. D. (2007). Self-regulation, ego depletion, and motivation. *Social and Personality Psychology Compass, 1*(1), 115–128.

Bem, D. J. (1972). Self-perception theory. *Advances in Experimental Social Psychology, 6*, 1–62.

Bischof, G., Freyer-Adam, J., Meyer, C., John, U., & Rumpf, H. J. (2012). Changes in drinking behavior among control group participants in early intervention studies targeting unhealthy alcohol use recruited in general hospitals and general practices. *Drug and Alcohol Dependence, 125*(1–2), 81–88.

Bitunjac, K., & Saraga, M. (2009). Alcohol intoxication in pediatric age: Ten-year retrospective study. *Croatian Medical Journal, 50*, 151–156.

Black, J. J., Tran, G. Q., Goldsmith, A. A., Thompson, R. D., Smith, J. P., & Welge, J. A. (2012). Alcohol expectancies and social self-efficacy as mediators of differential intervention outcomes for college hazardous drinkers with social anxiety. *Addictive Behaviors, 37*, 248–255.

Burton, D., Sussman, S., Hansen, W. B., Johnson, C. A., & Flay, B. R. (1989). Image attributions and smoking intentions among seventh grade students. *Journal of Applied Social Psychology, 19*, 656–664.

Caflisch, M., & Uldry, V. (2013). At the crossover of adolescent and alcohol. *Revue Medicale Suisse, 9*, 406–409.

Carey, K. B., Scott-Sheldon, L. A. J., Carey, M. P., & DeMartini, K. S. (2007). Individual-level interventions to reduce college student drinking: A meta-analytic review. *Addictive Behaviors, 32*, 2469–2494.

Champion, H. L., Foley, K. L., Durant, R. H., Hensberry, R., Altman, D., & Wolfson, M. (2004). Adolescent sexual victimization, use of alcohol and other substances, and other health risk behaviors. *Journal of Adolescent Health, 35*, 321–328.

Chassin, L., Presson, C. C., Sherman, S. J., Corty, E., & Olshavsky, R. W. (1981). Self-images and cigarette smoking in adolescence. *Personality and Social Psychology Bulletin, 7*(4), 670–676.

Chassin, L., Tetzloff, C., & Hershey, M. (1985). Self-image and social-image factors in adolescent alcohol use. *Journal of Studies on Alcohol, 46*(1), 39–47.

Cooper, M. L., Frone, M. R., Russell, M., & Mudar, P. (1995). Drinking to regulate positive and negative emotions: A motivational model of alcohol use. *Journal of Personality and Social Psychology, 69*, 990–1005.

Cox, W. M., & Klinger, E. (1988). A motivational model of alcohol use. *Journal of Abnormal Psychology, 97*(2), 168–180.

Cox, W. M., & Klinger, E. (2004). A motivational model of alcohol use: Determinants of use and change. In W. M. Cox & E. Klinger (Eds.), *Handbook of motivational counseling* (pp. 121–138). Wiley.

Cox, W. M., & Klinger, E. (2011). A motivational model of alcohol use: Determinants of use and change. In W. M. Cox & E. Klinger (Eds.), *Handbook of motivational counseling* (2nd ed., pp. 131–158). Wiley-Blackwell.

Demmel, R. (2003). *Motivational Interviewing: Ein Leitfaden für die Praxis*. Hogrefe.

Diestelkamp, S., Arnaud, N., Sack, P.-M., Wartberg, L., Daubmann, A., & Thomasius, R. (2014). Brief motivational intervention for adolescents treated for acute alcohol intoxication in the emergency department—A randomized-controlled trial. *BMC Emergency Medicine, 14*, 13.

Diestelkamp, S., Kriston, L., Arnaud, N., Wartberg, L., Sack, P.-M., Härter, M., & Thomasius, R. (2015). Drinking patterns of alcohol intoxicated adolescents in the emergency department: A latent class analysis. *Addictive Behaviors, 50*, 51–59.

Diestelkamp, S., Drechsel, M., Baldus, C., Wartberg, L., Arnaud, N., & Thomasius, R. (2016). Brief in person interventions for adolescents and young adults following alcohol-related events in emergency care: A systematic review and European evidence synthesis. *European Addiction Research, 22*, 17–35. https://doi.org/10.1159/000435877

Diestelkamp, S., Wartberg, L., Arnaud, N., & Thomasius, R. (2016). *Einfluss von Therapeuten- und Interventionsvariablen auf die Effektivität einer motivierenden Kurzintervention für Minderjährige nach akuter Alkoholintoxikation*. Praxis der Kinderpsychologie und Kinderpsychiatrie, *65*, 534–549.

Dilling, H., & Freyberger, H. J. (2001). *Taschenführer zur ICD-10. Klassifikation psychischer Störungen*. Huber.

Dimeff, L. A., Baer, J. S., Kivlahan, D. R., & Marlatt, G. A. (1999). *Brief alcohol screening and intervention for college students (BASICS). A harm reduction approach*. Guilford.

Earleywine, M., LaBrie, J. W., & Pedersen, E. R. (2008). A brief Rutgers alcohol problem index with less potential for bias. *Addictive Behaviours, 33*(9), 1249–1253.

Fandler, E., Scheer, P., Rödl, S., & Müller, W. (2008). Alkoholmissbrauch und –abhängigkeit bei Kindern und Jugendlichen. *Monatsschrift Kinderheilkunde, 156*, 591–604.

Fishbein, M., & Ajzen, I. (1975). *Belief, attitude, intention, and behavior: An introduction to theory and research*. Addison-Wesley.

Gesundheitsberichterstattung des Bundes. (2016). *Diagnosedaten der Krankenhäuser ab 2000; 2016. Aus dem Krankenhaus entlassene vollstationäre Patienten (einschl. Sterbe- und Stundenfälle) F10.0—Psychische und Verhaltensstörungen durch Alkohol—Akute Intoxikation (akuter Rausch) nach Wohnsitz, Alter und Geschlecht* [Fallzahl und je 100 000 Einwohner]. Retrieved 11 May, 2016, from http://www.gbe-bund.de.

Gibbons, F. X., Gerrard, M., & Lane, D. J. (2003). A social-reaction model of adolescent health risk. In J. M. Suls & K. A. Wallston (Eds.), *Social psychological foundations of health and illness* (pp. 107–136). Blackwell.

Groß, C., Mick, I., Reichert, J., & Zimmermann, U. S. (2016a). Adolescents admitted to in-patient treatment with alcohol intoxication: Risk and resilience factors associated with problematic alcohol use. *Journal of Alcoholism & Drug Dependence, 4*, 231. https://doi.org/10.4172/2329-6488.1000231

Groß, C., Reis, O., Kraus, L., Piontek, D., Zimmermann, U. S., & RISCA-Group. (2016b). Long-term outcomes after adolescent in-patient treatment due to alcohol intoxication: A control group study. *Journal of Alcoholism & Drug Dependence, 162*, 116–123.

Hampel, P., & Petermann, F. (2005). *SPS-J—Screening psychischer Störungen im Jugendalter. Deutschsprachige adaptation des Reynolds adolescent adjustment screening InventoryTM (RAASITM) von William M. Reynolds Gollwitzer*. Hogrefe.

Härter, M., Kentgens, M., Brandes, A., Bock, T., Dirmaier, J., & Erzberger, … Lambert, M. (2012). Rationale and content of psychenet: The Hamburg network for mental health. *European Archives of Psychiatry and Clinical Neuroscience, 262*(2), 57–63.

Havighurst, R. J. (1948). *Developmental tasks and education*. University of Chicago Press.

Healey, C., Rahmana, A., Faizal, M., & Kinderman, P. (2004). Underage drinking in the UK: Changing trends, impact and interventions. A rapid evidence synthesis. *International Journal of Drug Policy, 25*, 124–132.

Heather, N. (2014). Interpreting null findings from trials of alcohol brief interventions. *Frontiers in Psychiatry, 5*(85), 1–11. https://doi.org/10.3389/fpsyt.2014.00085

Heidenreich, T., & Hoyer, J. (2001). Stadien der Veränderung bei Substanzmissbrauch und -abhängigkeit: Eine methodenkritische Übersicht. *Sucht, 47*(3), 158–170.

Herring, R., Berridge, V., & Thom, B. (2008). Binge drinking: An exploration of a confused concept. *Journal of Epidemiology and Community Health, 62*, 476–479.

Hibell, B., Guttormsen, U., Ahlström, S., Balakireva, O., Bjarnason, T., Kokkevi, A., & Kraus, L. (2012). *The 2011 ESPAD report. Substance use among students in 36 European countries*. Retrieved 02 November, 2012, from http://www.espad.org/Uploads/ESPAD_reports/2011/The_2011_ESPAD_Report_FULL_2012_10_29.pdf.

IBM SPSS. (2011). New York.

Jessor, R. (1987). Problem-behavior theory, psychological development, and adolescent problem drinking. *British Journal of Addiction, 82*, 331–342.

Jessor, R. (1991). Risk behavior in adolescence: A psychological framework for understanding and action. *Journal of Adolescent Health, 12*, 597–605.

Jester, J. M., Wong, M. M., Cranford, J. A., Buu, A., Fitzgerald, H. E., & Zucker, R. A. (2015). Alcohol expectancies in childhood: Change with the onset of drinking and ability to predict adolescent drunkenness and binge drinking. *Addiction, 110*(1), 71–79.

Jordan, S., & Sack, P. M. (2009). Schutz- und Risikofaktoren. In R. Thomasius, M. Schulte-Markwort, U. J. Küstner, & P. Riedesser (Eds.), *Suchtstörungen im Kindes- und Jugendalter. Das Handbuch: Grundlagen und Praxis* (pp. 127–138). Schattauer.

Kaner, E. F., Dickinson, H. O., Beyer, F. R., Campbell, F., Schlesinger, C., Heather, N., Saunders, J. B., Burnand, B., & Pienaar, E. D. (2007). Effectiveness of brief alcohol interventions in primary care populations. *The Cochrane Database Systematic Reviews, 2*, CD004148. https://doi.org/10.1002/14651858.CD004148.pub3

Kraus, L., Hannemann, T.-V., Pabst, A., Müller, S., Kronthaler, F., Grübl, A., Stürmer, M., & Wolstein, J. (2013). Stationäre Behandlung von Jugendlichen mit akuter Alkoholintoxikation: Die Spitze des Eisbergs? *Gesundheitswesen, 75*, 456–464.

Kuntsche, E., Knibbe, R., Gmel, G., & Engels, R. (2005). Why do young people drink? A review of drinking motives. *Clinical Psychology Review, 25*(7), 841–861.

Kuttler, H. (2006). Hart am LimiT—HaLT: Ein Alkoholpraeventionsprojekt fuer Kinder und Jugendliche. *Suchtmedizin in Forschung und Praxis, 8*(1), 45–50.

Kuttler, H., Schwendemann, H., Reis, O., & Bitzer, E. M. (2016). Developmental hazards among young alcohol intoxicated patients. *Journal of Adolescent Health*, 1–9. https://doi.org/10.1016/j.jadohealth.2016.03.022

Kuzelová, M., Harárová, A., Ondriasová, E., Wawruch, M., Riedel, R., Benedeková, M., Kovács, L., & Plaková, S. (2009). Alcohol intoxication requiring hospital admission in children and adolescents: Retrospective analysis at the university children's hospital in the Slovak Republic. *Clinical Toxicology, 47*, 556–561.

Kypri, K., Langley, J. D., Saunders, J. B., & Cashell-Smith, M. L. (2007). Assessment may conceal therapeutic benefit: Findings from a randomized controlled trial for hazardous drinking. *Addiction, 102*(1), 62–70.

Laging, M. (2005). Assessment und Diagnostik in der sekundaeren Suchtpraevention bei Jugendlichen. *Praevention, 28*(1), 9–12.

Lang, S., & Kuttler, H. (2007). Projekt HaLT—Hart am LimiT. Frühintervention und kommunal verankerte Strategie zur Verhinderung von riskantem Rauschtrinken bei Kindern und Jugendlichen. *Wiener Zeitschrift für Suchtforschung, 30*(1), 27–37.

Lawson, P. J., & Flocke, S. A. (2009). Teachable moments for health behaviour change: A concept analysis. *Patient Education and Counseling, 76*, 25–3026.

Lee, M. R., Chassin, L., & Villalta, I. K. (2013). Maturing out of alcohol involvement: Transitions in latent drinking statuses from late adolescence to adulthood. *Development and Psychopathology, 25*(4 Pt 1), 1137–1153. https://doi.org/10.1017/S0954579413000424

Lim, S. S., Vos, T., Flaxman, A. D., Danaei, G., Shibuya, K., et al. (2012). A comparative risk assessment of burden of disease and injury attributable to 67 risk factors and risk factor clusters in 21 regions, 1990–2010: A systematic analysis for the global burden of disease study 2010. *The Lancet, 380*, 2224–2260.

Loukova, A. (2011). Study of acute alcohol poisoning in children admitted to an emergency hospital Pirogov in Sofia, Bulgaria. *Macedonian Journal of Medical Sciences, 4*, 275–280.

McBride, C. M., Emmons, K. M., & Lipkus, I. M. (2003). Understanding the potential of teachable moments: The case of smoking cessation. *Health Education Research, 18*(2), 156–170.

McCambridge, J., & Kypri, K. (2011). Can simply answering research questions change behaviour? Systematic review and meta-analysis of brief alcohol intervention trials. *PLoSOne, 6*(10), e23748. https://doi.org/10.1371/journal.pone.0023748

Miller, R. W. (1999). *Enhancing motivation for change in substance abuse treatment. Treatment improvement protocol (TIP) series 35*. U.S. Department of Health and Human Services.

Miller, R. W., & Rollnick, S. (2002). *Motivational interviewing. Preparing people for change*. Guilford.

Miller, R. W., & Rollnick, S. (2013). *Motivational interviewing. Preparing people for change*. Guilford.

Miller, R. W., & Rollnick, S. (2015). *Motivierende Gesprächsführung*. Lambertus.

Miller, W. R., & Rose, G. S. (2015). Motivational interviewing and decisional balance: Contrasting resposnes to client ambivalence. *Behavioural and Cognitive Psychotherapy, 43*, 129–141.

Miller, R. W., Zweben, D. S. W., DiClemente, C., & Rychtarik, R. G. (1995). Motivational enhancement therapy manual. In *NIAAA, project MATCH monograph series* (Vol. 2). NIAAA.

Monti, P. M., Colby, S. M., Barnett, N. P., Spirito, A., Rohsenow, D. J., Myers, M., Woolard, R., & Lewander, W. (1999). Brief intervention for harm reduction with alcohol-positive older adolescents in a hospital emergency department. *Journal of Consulting and Clinical Psychology, 67*, 989–994.

Monti, P. M., Barnett, N. P., Colby, S. M., Gwaltney, C. J., Spirito, A., Rohsenow, D. J., & Woolard, R. (2007). Motivational interviewing versus feedback only in emergency care for young adult problem drinking. *Addiction, 102*, 1234–1243.

Newcomb, M. D., & Bentler, P. M. (1989). Substance use and abuse among children and teenagers. *American Psychologist, 44*, 242–248.

Newton, A. S., Gokiert, R., Mabood, N., Ata, N., Dong, K., Ali, S., & Wild, T. C. (2013). Brief emergency department interventions for youth who use alcohol and other drugs: A systematic review. *Pediatric Emergengy Care, 29*(5), 673–684.

Nilsen, P., Baird, J., Mello, M., Nirenberg, T., Woolard, R., Bendtsen, P., & Longabaugh, R. (2008). A systematic review of emergency care brief alcohol interventions for injury patients. *Journal of Substance Abuse Treatment, 35*, 184–201.

Orford, J. (2001). Addiction as excessive appetite. *Addiction, 96*, 15–31.

Orth, B., & Töppich, J. (2015). *Der Alkoholkonsum Jugendlicher und junger Erwachsener in Deutschland 2014*. Ergebnisse einer aktuellen Repräsentativbefragung und Trends.

Prochaska, J. O., DiClemente, C. C., & Norcross, J. C. (1992). In search of how people change. Applications to addictive behaviors. *American Psychologist, 47*(9), 1102–1114.

Reis, O., Papke, M., & Haessler, F. (2009). Ergebnisse eines Projektes zur kombinierten Prävention jugendlichen Rauschtrinkens. *Sucht, 55*, 347–356.

Sack, P. M., Stolle, M., & Thomasius, R. (2009). *Erfassung alkoholintoxikierter Kinder und Jugendlicher bis 21 Jahre in Hamburg mittels eines Postkartenmeldesystems (E-AK21)*. Unveröffentlichter Forschungsbericht, Universitätsklinikum Hamburg-Eppendorf.

Sack, P. M., Diestelkamp, S., Küstner, U., & Thomasius, R. (2012). Gesundheitsnetz "Alkoholmissbrauch im Jugendalter": Verbesserung des Behandlungszugangs für Kinder und Jugendliche mit riskantem Alkoholkonsum. *Suchttherapie, 13*(1), 33–36.

Schmidt, C. S., Schulte, B., Seo, H. N., Kuhn, S., O'Donnell, A., Kriston, L., Verthein, U., & Reimer, J. (2016). Meta-analysis on the effectiveness of alcohol screening with brief interventions for patients in emergency care settings. *Addiction, 111*(5), 783–794.

Silbereisen, R., & Reese, A. (2001). Substanzgebrauch Jugendlicher: Illegale Drogen und Alkohol. In J. Raithel (Ed.), *Risikoverhaltensweisen Jugendlicher. Formen, Erklärungen und Prävention* (pp. 131–153). Leske und Budrich.

Sindelar, H. A., Barnett, N. P., & Spirito, A. (2004). Adolescent alcohol use and injury: A summary and critical review of the literature. *Minerva Pediatrica, 56*(3), 291–309.

Spirito, A., Monti, P. M., Barnett, N. P., Colby, S. M., Sindelar, H., Rohsenow, D. J., Lewander, W., & Myers, M. (2004). A randomized clinical trial of a brief motivational intervention for alcohol-positive adolescents treated in an emergency department. *Journal of Pediatrics, 145*, 396–402.

Spirito, A., Sindelar-Manning, H., Colby, S. M., Barnett, N. P., Lewander, W., Rohsenow, D. J., & Monti, P. M. (2011). Individual and family motivational interventions for alcohol-positive adolescents treated in an emergency department: Results of a randomized clinical trial. *Archives of Pediatrics and Adolescent Medicine, 165*, 269–274.

Steinberg, L. (2010). A dual systems model of adolescent risk-taking. *Developmental Psychobiology, 52*, 216–224.

Stolle, M., Sack, P.-M., & Thomasius, R. (2009). Rauschtrinken im Kindes- und Jugendalter. Epidemiologie, Auswirkungen und Intervention. *Deutsches Ärzteblatt, 106*(19), 323–328.

Stolle, M., Petersen, K. U., & Thomasius, R. (2010). *Antragsskizze zur Förderung des Projekts "Entwicklung und Evaluation eines Trainingsprogramms für Eltern suchtgefährdeter Kinder und Jugendlicher"*. Unveröffentlichte Antragsskizze, Universitätsklinikum Hamburg-Eppendorf.

Stolle, M., Sack, P. M., Broening, S., Baldus, C., & Thomasius, R. (2013). Brief intervention in alcohol intoxicated adolescent—A follow-up study in an access-to-care sample. *Journal of Alcoholism & Drug Dependence, 1*, 106. https://doi.org/10.4172/2329-6488.1000106

Strack, F., & Deutsch, R. (2004). Reflective and impulsive determinants of social behaviour. *Personality and Social Psychology Review, 8*, 220–247.

Stucki, C. (2002). *Die Therapiebeziehung differentiell gestalten. Intuitive Reaktionen, Patientenwahrnehmung und Beziehungsverhalten von Therapeuten in der Psychotherapie*. Universität Bern. Retrieved from http://www.zb.unibe.ch/download/eldiss/04stucki_c.pdf.

Swahn, M. H., Simon, T. R., Hammig, B. J., & Guerrero, J. L. (2004). Alcohol consumption behaviors and risk for physical fighting and injuries among adolescent drinkers. *Addictive Behaviors, 29*, 959–963.

Thomasius, R., Stappenbeck, J., Reis, O., Bilke-Hentsch, O., Sack, P.-M., & Hoch, E. (2016). Kinder und Jugendliche. Kap. 3.7.2. In K. Mann, E. Hoch, & A. Batra (Eds.), *S3-Leitlinie Screening, Diagnose und Behandlung alkoholbezogener Störungen* (pp. 129–142). Springer.

Tossmann, P., Kasten, L., Lang, P., & Strüber, E. (2009). Bestimmung der konkurrenten Validität des CRAFFT-d. Ein Screeninginstrument für problematischen Alkoholkonsum bei Jugendlichen. *Zeitschrift für Kinder- und Jugendpsychiatrie und Psychotherapie, 37*, 451–459.

Van Hoof, J. J., Van Der Lely, N., Pereira, R. R., & Van Dalen, W. E. (2010). Adolescent alcohol intoxication in the dutch hospital departments of pediatrics. *Journal of Studies on Alcohol and Drugs, 71*(3), 366–372.

Villa Schöpflin (2009). *Bundesmodellprojekt HaLT. Trainer-Manual und Projektdokumentation*. 3. Aufl. Lörrach: Villa Schöpflin. Retrieved 27 April, 2016, from http://www.halt-projekt.de/images/stories/pdf/handbuch_halt_2009.pdf.

Villa Schöpflin (2010). *Leitfaden und Gesprächswegweiser für das Brückengespräch*. Retrieved 27 April, 2016, from http://www.halt-projekt.de/images/stories/pdf/leitfaden_endfassung%2012.1.2010.pdf.

Viner, R. M., & Taylor, B. (2007). Adult outcomes of binge drinking in adolescence: Findings from a UK national birth cohort. *Journal of Epidemiology and Community Health, 61*, 902–907.

Wartberg, L., Kriston, L., Diestelkamp, S., Arnaud, N., & Thomasius, R. (2016). Factorial and criterion validity of the German version of the CRAFFT. *Addictive Behaviors, 59*, 42–47.

Wartberg, L., Diestelkamp, S., Arnaud, N., & Thomasius, R. (n.d.). *Einsatz des Screening-Instrumentes CRAFFT-d bei Jugendlichen, die wegen einer Alkoholintoxikation im Krankenhaus behandelt wurden*. Praxis der Kinderpsychologie und Kinderpsychiatrie.

West, R. (2013). *EMCDDA insights—Models of addiction*. European Monitoring Centre for Drugs and Drug Addiction. https://doi.org/10.2810/99994

Wiers, R. W., Bartholow, B. D., Van den Wildenberge, E., Thush, C., Engels, R. C. M. E., Sher, K. J., Grenard, J., Ames, S. L., & Stacy, A. W. (2007). Automatic and controlled processes and the development of addictive behaviors in adolescents: A review and model. *Pharmacology, Biochemistry and Behavior, 86*, 263–283.

Wiers, R. W., Ames, S. L., Hofmann, W., Krank, M., & Stacy, A. W. (2010). Impulsivity, impulsive and reflective processes and the development of alcohol use and misuse in adolescents and young adults. *Frontiers in Psychology, 1*(144), 1–12.

Wurdak, M., Lhle, K., Sturmer, M., Dirnberger, I., Fischer, U. C., Funk, T., Kraus, L., & Wolstein, J. (2013). Indikatoren für das Ausmaß jugendlichen Rauschtrinkens in Bayern. *Sucht, 59*(4), 225–233.

Wurdak, M., Wolstein, J., & Kuntsche, M. (2016). Effectiveness of a drinking-motive-tailored emergency-room intervention among adolescents admitted to hospital due to acute alcohol intoxication—A randomized controlled trial. *Preventive Medicine Reports, 3*, 83–89.

Yamada, S., Pepler, D., Jiang, D., Cappadocia, M. C., Craig, W., & Connolly, J. (2016). Developmental trajectories of adolescent substance use. *Journal of Child & Adolescent Substance Abuse, 25*(1), 33–48.

Yuma-Guerrero, P. J., Velasquez, M. M., von Sternberg, K., Maxson, T., & Garcia, N. (2012). Screening, brief intervention, and referral for alcohol use in adolescents: A systematic review. *Pediatrics, 130*(1), 115–122.

Index

R

S

T

V

W

Y

The manufacturer's authorised representative in the EU is Springer Nature Customer Service Centre GmbH, Europaplatz 3, 69115 Heidelberg, Germany. If you have any concerns regarding our products, please contact ProductSafety@springernature.com

Printed and bound by CPI Group (UK) Ltd, Croydon, CR0 4YY
30/09/2026
02225575-0020